PUBLIC HEALTH IN THE 21ST CENTURY

EFFECTIVE HEALTH COMMUNICATION FOR SUSTAINABLE DEVELOPMENT

PUBLIC HEALTH IN THE 21ST CENTURY

Additional books in this series can be found on Nova's website
under the Series tab.

Additional e-books in this series can be found on Nova's website
under the e-books tab.

PUBLIC HEALTH IN THE 21ST CENTURY

EFFECTIVE HEALTH COMMUNICATION FOR SUSTAINABLE DEVELOPMENT

PATCHANEE MALIKHAO

nova publishers
New York

Additional color graphics may be available in the e-book version of this book.

Library of Congress Cataloging-in-Publication Data

ISBN: 978-1-63484-807-7

Library of Congress Control Number: 2016936930

Published by Nova Science Publishers, Inc. † New York

With love and appreciation to
Foy & Nongluck Malikhao, my parents,
Gilbert Servaes & Alice Vandebergh, my in-laws,
and to
Jan, Fiona and Lisa Servaes, my family.

CONTENTS

List of Figures and Tables

Tables

Figures

ABBREVIATIONS

ABC	Abstinence, Be faithful and use a Condom
ADD	Attention Deficit Disorder
AIDS	Acquired Immunodeficiency Syndrome
BCC	Behavioral Change Communication
BMI	Body Mass Index
BSE	Bovine Spongiform Encephalopathy
bST	Bovine Samatotropin
CBO	Community Based Organization
CDC	Centers for Disease Control
CFC	Chlorofluorocarbons
CIC	Community Information Center
COPD	Chronic Obstructive Pulmonary Disease
DI	Diffusion Index
DNA	DeoxyriboNucleic Acid
EPA	United States Environmental Protection Agency
GI	Glycemic Index
GIS	Geographic Information System
GL	Glycemic Loads
GNP	Gross National Product
HBM	Health Belief Model
HDI	Human Development Index
HHS	US Department of Health and Human Services
HIV	Human Immunodeficiency Virus
HPV	Human Papillomavirus
HUD	US Department of Housing and Urban Development
IBM	Integrated Behavioral Model
ICT	Information and Communication Technologies
IEC	Information, Education, and Communication
IFJ	International Federation of Journalists
IFRC	International Federation of Red Cross and Red Crescent Societies
IMF	International Monetary Fund
KAP	Knowledge, Attitude, and Practice
LGBT	Lesbian, Gay, Bi-sexual, Transgender

MCA	Multiple Correspondence Analysis
MCP	Multicultural Policies
MDGs	Millennial Development Goals
M&E	Monitoring and Evaluation
MERS	Middle East Respiratory Syndrome
MSC	Most Significant Change
NCD	Non-Communicable Disease
NGO	Non-Governmental Organization
OECD	Organization for Economic Co-operation and Development
PAPM	Precaution Adoption Process Model
PAR	Participatory Action Research
PCB	Polychlorinated biphenyls
PLA	Participatory Learning and Action
PLWHA	People Living with HIV/AIDS
PR	Participatory Research
PRECEDE	Predisposing, Reinforcing, and Enabling Constructs in Educational/Environmental Diagnosis
PROCEED	Policy, Regulatory, and Organizational Constructs in Educational and Environmental Development
RSS	Rich Site Summary
PSA	Public Service Announcement
SARS	Severe Acute Respiratory Syndrome
SDGs	Sustainable Development Goals
SES	Socio-economic Status
SC	Significant Change
SCT	Social Cognitive Theory
SDT	Self-Determination Theory
SIDS	Sudden Infant Death Syndrome
SLT	Social Learning Theory
SSHRC	Social Sciences and Humanities Research Council
STD	Sexually Transmitted Diseases
STI	Sexually Transmitted Infections
TB	Tuberculosis
TRA	Theory of Reasoned Action
TPB	Theory of Planned Behavior
TTM	Trans Theoretical Model
UGC	User Generated Content
UNDP	United Nations Development Programme
UNFPA	United Nations Population Fund
URL	Uniform Resource Locator
vCJD	Variant Creutzfeldt-Jakob Disease
WB	World Bank
WHO	World Health Organization
WWW	World Wide Web

FOREWORD

Health communication promoted in this book is based on a participatory model underpinned by the multiplicity paradigm. Strategies suggested in this book are practical examples to encourage the reader to design his/her own strategies to serve a particular community. Before one can devise a strategy for health promotion and disease prevention, one needs to understand that a top-down communication approach cannot change nor sustain people's health behaviors. On the contrary, one needs to create an enabling environment or a context that supports an individuals' decision to change their behavior. How to achieve sustainability in health or health for all, that's what this book hopes to achieve. We will try to guide the reader through eight chapters plus a conclusion section.

Chapter one elucidates concepts such as health, wellness, well-being, and health communication. History of health communication will be explained as well as sustainable development, which incorporates the elements of health communication in its goals.

Chapter two explores all health communication theories currently being used, and analyzes them in relation to development paradigms. The multiplicity paradigm and its components will be explained at length as the framework of participatory-based communication about/on health.

Chapter three teases out the impact of globalization on individual and community health and diseases. The relationship between sustainability and health will be illuminated.

Chapter four focuses on the context of health. Biosocial, geosocial, socioeconomic, cultural, and environmental factors that contribute to health inequalities will be elucidated. This chapter, as well as chapter three, is important for health communicators to be aware of possible obstacles in communicating on/about health.

Chapter five discusses intercultural communication and how to bring about sustainability in health. Health communication for sustainable development, under the framework of the multiplicity paradigm, will be the highlight of this chapter.

Chapter six introduces the reader to the tools for health communication for sustainability. Thus, traditional as well as new media will be explored.

Chapter seven illuminates the principles of devising health communication strategies for sustainability.

Chapter eight builds on chapter seven. It provides practical advice and examples of strategies needed to improve health through a life course to empower people; tackle communicable, non-communicable diseases, and provide all necessary supportive systems to maintain and sustain a healthy community where everyone is included.

Finally, the conclusion summarizes this holistic approach to health communication. It emphasizes that a health communicator must engage people in the community from a multiplicity perspective. He or she possess intercultural communication competency, media literacy, health literacy, capacity building competency, media technology skills, and understands participatory-based health communication strategies. Apart from that, social and environmental determinants of health should not be ignored. The health communicator must be creative and able to devise strategies that suit a particular community.

Please keep in mind that communication strategies suggested in this book are just examples to inspire you to come up with your own strategies more suitable to your community. I am sure that there are a lot of strategies out there, thanks to innovations in media technology, that add to a wealth of creative ideas. Be inspired and be creative.

Enjoy reading!

With best wishes,

Patchanee Malikhao
Hong Kong, February 23rd, 2016.

ACKNOWLEDGMENTS

I had thought of writing a book on health communication since I resided in Amherst, Massachusetts, USA. An outline was written and announced at an International Conference in Boston. But I discarded the plan because it was not what I really wanted, as it was not for sustainability. The idea of integrating sustainability with health communication came back when I arrived in Hong Kong, and read many interesting books that inspired me to think about these topics again. I proposed the outline to Nova Science Publishers, Inc. in New York, and it was accepted within two weeks. Here is the book that I am very proud to present to you.

I would like to thank Nova Science Publishers, Inc. for publishing this book, which is my second single-author book. I would also like to thank the following publishers and authors who granted me permission to reprint their figures:

1) Chin Saik Yoon, Southbound Publishers, Penang, Malaysia for Figure I: "The Behavior Development and Change Model," from Carnegie, R., McKee, N., Dick, B., Reitemeier, P. et al. (2000: 162). Making Change Possible: Creating an Enabling Environment. In (N. McKee, E. Manoncourt, S.Y. Chin, and R. Carnegie eds.) *Involving People Evolving Behavior*. Penang: Southbound.
2) Jan Servaes, for Figure 2: "A Communication Model with Active Social Participation," from: Servaes, J. (1999: 90). Communication for Development. One world, multiple cultures. Cresskill, NJ: Hampton Press Inc.
3) The University of Rochester Press, for Figure 3: "The Self-Determination Model of Patients' Motivation Behavior, and Health," from Williams, G. G. (2002: 240). Improving Patient's Health Through Supporting the Autonomy of Patients and Providers. In (E. L. Deci & R. M. Ryan eds.) *Handbook of Self-Determination Research*. Rochester, NY: the University of Rochester Press, pp. 233-254.
4) John Wiley and sons, Inc. for Figure 4: "PRECEDE-PROCEED Planning Model," from Gielen, A. C., McDonald, E. M., Gary, T. L. & Bone, L. R. (2008: 410). Using the PRECEDE-PROCEED Model to Apply Health Behavior Theories. In *Health Behavior and Health Education. Theory, Research, and Practice*. (4th ed.) (Eds. K. Glanz, B. K. Rimer & K. Viswanath). San Francisco, CA: Jossey-Bass, pp. 407-433. And for Figure 5: "Ecological Model of Four Domains of Active Living," from Sallis, J. F., Cervero, R. B., Ascher, W., Henderson, K. A., Kraft, M.K., and Kerr, J.

(2006). “An Ecological Approach to Creating More Physically Active Communities.” Annual Review of Public Health, 27, 297-322.

5) Oxfam International, UK. for Figure 6: “A safe and just space for humanity to thrive in: a first illustration,” from Raworth, K. (2012). A Safe and Just Space for Humanity. Can we live within the doughnut? Oxfam Discussion Papers, p. 4 https://www.oxfam.org/sites/www.oxfam.org/files/dp-a-safe-and-just-space-for-humanity-130212-en.pdf, accessed January 20th, 2016.

Last but not least, I would like to thank the City University of Hong Kong Library for their good resources without which I could not have accomplished this task.

I have learned a lot while writing this book. I hope that the reader also learns something while reading it.

Thank you so much for your support and interest.

Chapter 1

HISTORY AND DISCOURSES OF HEALTH COMMUNICATION AND SUSTAINABLE DEVELOPMENT

ABSTRACT

This chapter discusses discourses on health, illness, wellness, and well-being. The importance of communicating well on health will be explained and why "health communication" has become a special discipline will be illuminated. The history of health communication and roles that health communication plays in the prevention and curation of diseases will be investigated. The highlight of this chapter is the link of health communication to sustainable development. Development, sustainable development and development paradigms will be explained in relation to health communication.

Keywords: health, illness, wellness, well-being, health communication, development, sustainability, sustainable development

INTRODUCTION

"Good health underpins social and economic development and strengthens policies across all sectors" (WHO Europe 2013: 11). Good health is related to the success of both economic and social development of a nation. Poor health among citizens weakens efficient human resources and productivity; and thereby decreases tax revenues and economic growth, social cohesion, down to individual personhood[1], and well-being. Good health is seen as a human right and equity among peoples.

WHAT CONSTITUTES HEALTH?

"Health" is an open concept which requires a holistic approach to address. Health determinants can be social, ecological and personal. Already in 1946 the World Health

[1] Janzen (2002: 148) defines personhood as the self-conscious yet social identity of individuals.

Organization (WHO, 1946) acknowledged the multiple dimensions of health, and defined health as "more than the absence of disease."

The constitution of the World Health Organization (WHO, 2006) states clearly:

> Health is a state of complete physical, mental and social well-being and not merely the absence of disease or infirmity.
> The enjoyment of the highest attainable standard of health is one of the fundamental rights of every human being without distinction of race, religion, political belief, economic or social condition.
> The health of all peoples is fundamental to the attainment of peace and security and is dependent upon the fullest co-operation of individuals and States.
> The achievement of any State in the promotion and protection of health is of value to all.
> Unequal development in different countries in the promotion of health and control of disease, especially communicable disease, is a common danger.
> Healthy development of the child is of basic importance; the ability to live harmoniously in a changing total environment is essential to such development.
> The extension to all peoples of the benefits of medical, psychological and related knowledge is essential to the fullest attainment of health.
> Informed opinion and active co-operation on the part of the public are of the utmost importance in the improvement of the health of the people.
> Governments have a responsibility for the health of their peoples which can be fulfilled only by the provision of adequate health and social measures.

This definition elucidates that health development is a desirable goal for any society, and everyone has the right to a healthy life. To live a healthy life concerns many aspects, such as wellness, well-being, morality, human values, spirituality, and the absence of infirmity. Wellness is related to an individual's abilities to function to his/her full potential (Dunn 1977: 9-16); it is somewhat overlapping with well-being. Well-being is related to human values and morality to maintain good mental health and spirituality (Harris 2010: 34, Hunter et al. 2013: 197). Health can be seen as a means of attaining human well-being. Not only does a healthy person have a functional physical body, s/he also possesses healthy psycho-social characteristics to maintain good relationships with others. Health and illness are not entirely separate concepts; health fits in a continuum of death and optimal wellness, with death at one end and optimal wellness at the other (Sarafino 2006: 2).

Janzen (2002: 69) explains why the definition of health as absence of disease, disability, pain and discomfort is not appropriate because aging, fatigue, birth impairs, and growth disorder can be included as disease as well. Pain cannot be categorized as disease as it can be a part of a life course such as teething, menstruation and childbirth. Certain conditions that are disabling, such as pregnancy or baby's inability to do certain acts like adults, are not diseases either.

Thus, being healthy does not mean only being free from diseases and disparity but implies the ability to manage them. It is important that one lives in a good environment. To have a good environment is the effort of a community to maintain and sustain the health of its members. Factors that contribute to a good environment can be socio-economic-politico-ecological-cultural as well as bio-medical. Dimensions of health are listed in Table 1.1.

Table 1.1. Dimensions of health, wellness and well-being

Physical—fitness, flexibility, strength, agility, and other physical indices such as muscle tone, body mass index, cholesterol level, and blood pressure. Models often focus on health – behaviors and the actions needed to support health, such as self-care, lifestyle and preventive medicine. **Psychological/emotional**—positive attitudes, realistic self-esteem and optimism, awareness of feeling, and resilience. **Intellectual/cognitive**—the ability to learn, be creative, think critically and other higher order cognitive skills. **Spiritual**—a person's values and beliefs, a sense of meaning and purpose in life, inner peace, and an ability to transcend the personal self. **Occupational**—the optimal use of one's skills for meaningful and satisfying activities and work, which may be paid or unpaid. Recreational activities and environment. **Environment**—self-mastery and able to manage one's life; or an understanding of the importance of the environment on an individual's health.

Source: Hunter, J., Marshall, J., Corcoran and K., Leeder, S. (2013). A Positive Concept of Health—Interviews with Patients and Practitioners in an Integrative Medicine Clinic. Complementary Therapies in Clinical Practice 19 (2013) 197-203, p. 198.

Table 1.2. A matrix with four dimensions of health literacy applied to three health domains

	Access/obtain information relevant to health	Understand information relevant to health	Process/appraise information relevant to health	Apply/use information relevant to health
Healthcare	Ability to access information on medical or clinical issues	Ability to understand medical information and derive meaning	Ability to interpret and evaluate medical information	Ability to make informed decision on medical issues
Disease prevention	Ability to access information on risk factors for health	Ability to understand information on risk factors and derive meaning	Ability to interpret and evaluate information on risk factors for health	Ability to make informed decision on risk factors for health
Health promotion	Ability to update oneself on determinants of health in the social and physical environment	Ability to understand information on determinants of health in the social and physical environment and derive meaning	Ability to interpret and evaluate information on health determinants in the social and physical environment	Ability to make informed decisions on health determinants in the social and physical environment

Source: Sorensen, K., Van den Broucke, S., Fullam, J., Doyle, G., et al. (2012). Health Literacy and Public Health: A Systematic Review and Integration of Definitions and Models. BMC Public Health, 12:80, p.10 of 13. http://www.biomedcentral.com/1471-2458/12/80.

From Table 1.1, health of a person is a broad domain covering many indicators. A lack or incomplete fulfillment in each of these domains will result in unhealthy life or even sickness.

Indicators of health status of a nation are measured by infant mortality, prenatal care services, obesity rate, life expectancy, homicide and suicide rate, hypertension prevalence, income of the population (Spector 2000: 12). Another indicator of health status of an individual or a nation is the concept of "health literacy." Although the definition of health literacy is quite diverse, Sorensen et al. (2012: 9/13) reviewed literature and came up with a matrix with 12 dimensions of health literacy as illustrated in Table 1.2.

From Table 1.2, health literacy is seen as a process toward quality of life that requires cognitive, behavioral, and societal skills and abilities including communication and intercultural communication competences to achieve autonomy and self-empowerment toward desirable health behavior change for sustainability (Sorensen et al. 2012: 10). In order to support and sustain change of behavior, communication as a process of understanding and sharing meaning is the key (Schiavo 2007: 6-7). Communicating about health behaviors is not only the task of public health specialists. It involves every conscious human being: patients; doctors; stakeholders in a community: adolescents, adults, senior citizens, caregivers, social activists, health campaign managers, religious leaders, local authorities; and others. Communicating about health is indeed intercultural as it concerns communicating within and among people from different races, cultures, ages, languages, abilities, sexual orientations, gender, social class, education levels, religions, worldviews, and beliefs. Communicating about health also requires multi-disciplinary teamwork: anthropologists, sociologists, linguists, mass communication and new media reporters, public health professionals, healthcare providers, economists, social market analysts, public relations specialists, media advocates, social science researchers, and stakeholders with local wisdom.

What Is Health Communication?

Health communication encompasses intrapersonal, interpersonal, group, organizational, and societal communication. However, the definition of health communication varies.

We refer to a few mainstream definitions used by many health communication scholars. First, Lederman (2010: 236) sees it from the social interpretation and audience-centered perspective. She emphasizes the role that communication plays to define health and wellness, illness and disease, as well as to develop strategies to tackle health-related issues. Second, Seidman, Silberg, and Patrick's (2013: 180) definition is similar to Lederman's but focuses more on the hardware or the technology of communications and the educational strategies. These two definitions view communication as a top-down or communicator-centered perspective. Next, Dutta and Zoller (2008: 3) categorize the health communication scholarship into two perspectives: a process-based approach, which concerns social interpretation via symbolic interaction; and a message-based perspective, which concerns the creation of effective health messages and communication strategies to involve stakeholders. This viewpoint is still very close to a top-down and one-way communication mainstream.

Schiavo's (2007: 7) definition is quite different. Schiavo (2007: 7), arguing that health communication is a multifaceted and multidisciplinary approach, emphasizes the sharing of health-related information to diverse sorts of audience with the aims to influence or support health behavior or policy that will improve health behavior. This view of health communication pays much attention to the engagement of the stakeholders and their influences to the implementation in a bottom-up perspective. Thus, in Schiavo's perspective, the communication process is a two-way street.

Development and health are closely related. The population cannot reach the highest potentials of collaborative endeavor without possessing the physical and mental strength of individuals necessary for development work and social change (Prasad 2009 b: 362). Lie and Servaes (2015: 245) report that health communication is the most developed sub-discipline in the field of Communication for Development and Social Change and has been covered in many publications under the theme of Communication for Development. The health communication for sustainable development concept advocated in this book is *the art and technique of motivating and involving people to improve on health status, health disparities, health literacy, health information and knowledge of themselves or of their community and influencing on the healthcare policies of their community*. It is more than just a two-way communication process but also context-oriented and interdisciplinary-based. This means, an interdisciplinary study by which all stakeholders are engaged in a participatory-based advocacy process, underpinned by the social determinants of health, to devise their own strategies to improve the health of individuals and communities (Servaes & Malikhao 2009). In order to achieve long-term goals of health for all, top-down, bottom-up, and horizontal (by way of participating or peer-to-peer) approaches must be integrated for planning and implementation. That involves five approaches of communication:

a) Behavior change communication through mainly interpersonal communication,
b) Mass communication such as community media, mass media, and new media via Information and Communication Technologies (ICTs),
c) Advocacy communication, which is comprised of interpersonal and/or mass communication,
d) Participatory communication, which is comprised of interpersonal communication and community media, and
e) Communication for structural and sustainable social change, which consists of interpersonal communication, participatory communication, and mass communication (Servaes & Malikhao 2009).

Each communication strategy may influence different levels of health outcomes. The mass media may improve on the knowledge about health behavior, health issues, disease and prevention or have an impact on the positive attitude toward health behavior. Personal media can help in changing health behavior. As good health communication projects need funding and support, advocacy communication is very important to secure approval from sponsors or policy makers. Participatory-based advocacy engages the stakeholders to voice and take control of the health issues in their community to the policy makers. Effective health communication requires that the policy and planning and strategic communication about health should be defined by the people and for the people in the community so that the community achieves sustainability on health or health equity.

History and Trends of Health Communication

Health communication emerged as an area of study in its own right in the late 1950s in the US. Before that, it was part of the health education and training in the medical and public health areas. Actually, it can be traced back to the eighteenth- and nineteenth-century public health campaigns promoting hygiene and immunization (Wallington 2014: 169).

As most of the emerging mass media and communication research in the late 40s and early 50s built on the modernization paradigm (will be discussed more in detail in *Chapter 2*), communication theories and models used in health-related research were developed from the field of social psychology and sociology. An important study that lead to the development of the formation of a theory called the "Health Belief Model" widely used in health communication stems from a tuberculosis (TB) screening study in 1959 (Kar, Alcalay & Alex 2001: 50). The Health Belief Model or HBM has been used until now in health education and for the promotion of health behavior. The model adopted the learning theories derived from the Stimulus-Response Theory and Cognitive Theory (Rimer 2008: 47). These theories were used to explain inter- and intrapersonal communication in communication studies. Moreover, interpersonal communication theories, such as persuasion, adopted from social psychology, have been used to ensure desirable health outcomes. Theories and practices in health education and health behavior, together with interpersonal communication, group, and organizational communication theories, were in fashion since the development of the Diffusion of Innovations in communication studies by Rogers in 1962. Rogers' model combines rural sociology, medical sociology, communication studies, and marketing (Oldenburg & Glaz 2008: 314-315). Many health-related studies from the 1950s to the 1970s focused on disease prevention, behavior change interventions, health promotion, drugs and tobacco prevention (Kar, Alcalay & Alex 2001: 50-54). In the 1970s, organization and societal communication were introduced in family planning communication studies through the "Stage Theories in Behavior Change." They integrated knowledge in social psychology, communication, marketing and advertising, social marketing, psychotherapy, and family planning and reproductive health (Melkote & Steeves 2001: 129-130).

Lupton (1994: 56) reports that the term, "health communication," started being widely used in the 1980s and early 1990s. In the United Kingdom, the meaning of health communication had largely been focused on patient and health care provider communication (Lupton 1994: 56). However, in the United States and Australia the meaning had been expanded to include health education, health promotion, preventive medicine, organizational communication, and interpersonal communication in the health care setting (Irwin 1989: 32-40). Later on in the 2000s new communication technology, linguistics, medical sociology, medical anthropology and ecological studies were integrated in the field of health communication.

Contemporary health communication synthesizes six trends of disciplines: communication studies; human behavior and relations research; action research for health and human services program development around the world; the flourish of schools of public health starting from 1910s; the funding for prevention programs and agenda setting initiated by nonprofit and governmental institutions; and the mushrooming of targeted health promotion communication campaigns (Kar, Alacalay & Alex 2011: 46, 56).

The mainstream health communication studies in the US are mainly in the cybernetic tradition of information processing, and in the socio-psychological tradition of dealing with cognitive, emotional, and behavioral effects. Quantitative data are collected through the Health Belief Model and/or the Theory of Reasoned Action, Theory of Planned Behavior, or Integrated Behavioral Model (will be discussed in detail in *Chapter 2*). That can be studied at intrapersonal and interpersonal levels of communication. The combination of interpersonal and organizational communication theories, such as the PRECEDE- PROCEED model or the organizational change theory, are dominant in the area of health promotion.

While ecological models, highlighting the importance of the context in which health communication takes place, emerged in the 1950s (Sallis, Own & Fisher 2008: 468), it lasted until the 1970s before the socio-cultural environment became fully addressed in health communication studies (Sharf & Vanderford 2003: 9). Nowadays qualitative health communication studies cover a wide range going from the rhetorical tradition or shared common meaning; the semiotic tradition or communication as intersubjective mediation by signs and sign systems; the phenomenological tradition or communication as dialogue or experience of otherness; the sociocultural tradition or communication as a symbolic process that produces and reproduces shared sociocultural patterns; up to the critical tradition that applies critical theory to health and illness (Babrow & Matson 2003: 47-53).

From these accounts, we can see that health communication has come afar from merely bio-medical interventions. It concerns the individuals, the socials, and the ecology. The study area spans over health equity, healthcare, health disparities, social support, life and illness narratives, the role of language and culture in health disparities, health experiences such as end of life experiences, body and communication, therapeutic relationships, community-based communication, new media and information, and communication technologies and health, etc.

In sum, health communication calls for a diversity and integration of theories, methodologies, analyses, and strategies to engage and empower the locals to act upon their own- and community health. That is one of the goals of development: *health for all.*

Development Is Also a Discourse

Scholars and ordinary people alike talk about "development" so much that it has become a cliché. The term "development" emerged after the Second World War when the world was divided into the part that needed reconstruction from damages caused by the war, and the other part that was former colonies, which may not have been damaged from the war but needed to catch up with the rest of the "developed" world (Payutto 2003: 10). The term "undeveloped" was used then for those countries in the second category, but later on it was eulogized to "less-developed" and "developing" in the late 1960s (Payutto 2003: 11).

In the 1960s, development meant material growth. At the individual level, it meant how much money one could make; a house and a car (at least), and more. At the national level, it meant many roads, railroads, airports; high gross national products (GNP)/gross domestic products (GDP); electricity everywhere; high literacy rates; wide-coverage communications, wide-coverage mass communication (there was no internet access yet). At that time development concerned only the economic dimension: growth in terms of GNP and per capita income. This notion of development is still used till now, but there have been many more social and human rights indicators added to this economic aspect of development. Putting the emphasis on infrastructure building and money making alone did not solve problems of income distribution or a fair share of services for the "underserved" in society. The phrase "modernized but not developed" is coined with this kind of society; a society equipped with modern infrastructure but where social injustice abounds: be it discrimination, social disintegration, gaps in opportunities and social capital, unequal healthcare and services etc. Social justice concerns mitigating and eventually eradicating poverty and illiteracy, upholding human rights, having sound environmental policy, equity for opportunities and quality of life for healthy personal and social development (Levy & Sidel 2006: 8). Social injustice occurs when a country is claimed developed by an indicator that people mistook modernization for development.

Development should also mean the safety of life, a safety net for the underserved, and income distribution, the ability of the locals to organize and vitalize or revitalize their own community, as Wolfgang Sachs (2013: 5) puts it:

> On the one hand there are those who implicitly identify development with economic growth, calling for more relative equity in GDP. Their use of the word "development" reinforces the hegemony of the economic worldview… On the other hand, there are those who identify development with more rights and resources for the poor and powerless. Their use of the word calls for de-emphasizing growth in favor of greater autonomy of communities.

One can see that development is indeed a discourse; the meaning of it is up to one's interpretation. For P. A. Payutto, a renowned Buddhist scholar from Thailand, development from within or human development should come first. According to Payutto, greed (lobha), hatred (dosa) and ditthi (a domain comprising the following subsets: worldview, ideology, beliefs, religious beliefs and social values) are three root causes of the environmental crisis and shortage of resources. According to him (Payutto 2007: 55-63), the beliefs or ditthi that hold control of world civilization can be categorized into three groups, as follows:

a) The perception that mankind is separable from nature and can control or manipulate nature. Hence, the construction of dams, encroachment of forests, leaving carbon footprints, etc. are symbolic representations of this belief.
b) The perception that fellow human beings are not "fellow human beings." Hence, slavery, modern day slavery such as child labor, migrant labor, forced prostitution, human trafficking, the demolition of the Native Americans or the aborigines in Australia in the past, and racial discrimination in many parts of the world.
c) The perception that happiness relies on material wealth possessions. This is one of the dimensions of development as growth already explained. This can create an issue of the haves discriminating against the have-nots.

Under these views, people developed their lifestyles in a violent, hostile and competitive environment. Technology development for controlling nature or for aiding humans is a double-edged sword. Lifestyle aided by technology makes new generations more sedentary than its ancestors. Material wealth acquisition without caring about the fellow human beings causes exploitation and clusters of wealth. The socio-economic divide between the haves and the have-nots can cause social illnesses (such as drug abuses, AIDS, suicides, violence, to name a few), individual illnesses (such as stress, mental illness, communicable diseases such as Avian Influenza, SARS, mad cow disease etc.), and non-communicable diseases (such as diabetes, obesity, and cardiovascular diseases). The change of lifestyle for economic reasons for people from developing countries to developed ones also causes changes in genes, due to the interplay of the bio-medical and social environment, and resulting in so-called Western diseases (such as cancer, diabetes, cardiovascular diseases etc.) (Pollard 2008).

Sustainable Development: What Does That Mean?

From a Western perspective, sustainable development is "development that meets the needs of the present without compromising the ability of future generations to meet their own needs" (Brundtland Commission 1987). Vague it may sound but according to many scholars this concept should include economic, social, ecological and cultural dimensions. The movement for sustainability, according to Cox and Pezzullo (2016: 264), concerns three Es: Environmental protection, Economic health, and Equity (social justice), and three Ps: People, Prosperity, and the Planet. In other words, sustainability does not only concern a commitment to the environment, but also to social justice and economic well-being.

Sustainable development should at least address five areas: water and sanitation; energy; human health; agricultural productivity; and biodiversity and ecosystem management. As health disparities are related to race, ethnicity, gender, income, education, sexual orientation, quality of care, or geography (Wallington 2014: 170), health communication should be considered a part of communication for development to tackle these disparities and improve on healthcare in order to achieve health equity.

The pursuit of sustainability requires a participatory political system that allows citizens to make decisions by themselves; an economic system that provides equity and social justice; a production system that conserves the ecology; a technological system that cultivates fair trade and finance; an administrative system that is flexible and is self-correcting; and a communication system that gets the above-mentioned organized and accepted by all stakeholders in the society (Servaes 2013: 4).

Sustainability, as identified by the UN under the Millennium Development Goals (MDG), aims to

- Eliminating extreme poverty and hunger;
- Achieving universal primary education;
- Promoting gender equality and empowering women;
- Reducing child mortality;
- Improving maternal health;
- Combating HIV/AIDS, malaria, and other diseases;
- Ensuring environmental sustainability; and
- Developing a global partnership for development (United Nations 2008).

At the time of writing this book (in 2015), all of the above-mentioned health items are still ongoing issues. No sustainability has been achieved yet. Perhaps, it is therefore about time contemplating on the strategies used and considering on how to approach sustainability from another perspective.

For an Eastern perspective, P.A. Payutto states that cooperation and harmony should be the goals for sustainability (Payutto 2007: 61-66). According to Payutto (1998: 168-173), sustainability involves ecology, economy and evolvability. The term "evolvability" means the potential of human beings to develop themselves into less selfish persons. A developed human being should be free from five covetousness or possessiveness (macchariya) which are:

- Possessiveness or avarice of locality and country;
- Possessiveness or avarice of group and family, including ethnic and religious groups;
- Possessiveness or avarice of material wealth;
- Possessiveness or avarice of class or caste, including social standing, skin color, and so on.
- Possessiveness or avarice of knowledge and learning, including intellectual achievements and attainments (Payutto 2007: 67).

Arguing that the terms "human rights" and "religious tolerance" stem from historical backgrounds of division, segregation, and competition in the West, Payutto prefers to discuss freedom from three perspectives: as physical freedom, which is freedom from want and deprivation of four basic needs; as social freedom, which is freedom from being exploited from others; and most importantly, as inner freedom, which is the ability to be contented without exploiting fellow human beings or nature (Payutto 2007: 66-70). Inner freedom is the foundation for physical and social freedom. In other words, human development or development from within must come first. An Eastern interpretation of sustainable development combines an economic balance with human development.

Conclusion

Health Communication for Sustainable Development: Yes, It Is Possible!

Health literacy and health for all are goals for sustainable development. Health literacy can be a symbolic representation of inner freedom. Health for all can stand for social freedom, social justice and equity. To achieve these goals, communication strategies are needed. Health communication requires both a quantitative and qualitative approach to study it. Good bio-medical research is a foundation for good in-depth social interpretative research to explicate the social determinants that may hinder or support health outcomes. The most important thing for health communication study and research is a suitable theoretical framework that sees health holistically. Life is not just about quantifiable variables and numbers. There should be room for interpretation from a Social Interpretation point of view and the application of multiple and mixed research methodologies in order to reach realistic and effective outcomes. In other words, there is no need to spend time and money on research for the sake of showing the statistical competence of the researchers, as seems to be the case in too many health communication projects. That leads to the study of theories in *Chapter 2*.

REFERENCES

Babrow, A. S. & Mattson, M. (2003). Theorizing about Health Communication. In Handbook of Health Communication. (Eds. T. L. Thompson, A. Dorsey, K. I. Miller, and R. Parrot). New York-London: Lawrence Erlbaum Associates, Inc., pp. 35-61.

Brundtland, G. H. & World Commission on Environment and Development. (1987). *Our Common Future* (vol. 383). Oxford: Oxford University Press.

Chan, M. (2013). Foreword. In *Health 2020. A European Policy Framework and Strategy for the 21st Century*. Copenhagen: World Health Organization (WHO) Regional Office for Europe, pp. 8.

Dutta, M. & Zoller, H. (2008). Theoretical Foundations. Interpretive, Critical, and Cultural Approaches to Health Communication. In Emerging Perspectives in Health Communication. Meaning, Culture, and Power. (Eds., H. M. Zoller and M. J. Dutta). New York and London: Routledge, pp. 1-27.

Harris, S. (2010). *The Moral Landscape. How Science Can Determine Human Values*. New York-London-Toronto-Sydney: Free Press.

Human Development Report (2010). *The Real Wealth of Nations*. New York: United Nations Development Program. http: hdr.undp.org/en/media/HDR_2010_EN_Complete_reprint.pdf (accessed 21 June 2013).

Hunter, J., Marshall, J., Corcoran, K. and Leeder, S. (2013). A Positive Concept of Health—Interviews with Patients and Practitioners in an Integrative Medicine Clinic. *Complementary Therapies in Clinical Practice* 19, 197-203. http://dx.doi.org/10.1016/j.ctcp.2013.07.001.

Irwin, H. (1989). Health Communication: The research agenda. *Media Information Australia*. 54, pp. 32-40.

Janzen, J.M. (2002). *The Social Fabric of Health: An Introduction to Medical Anthropology*. Boston: McGrawHill.

Kar, S. B., Alcalay, R. & Alex, S. (2001). The Evolution of Health Communication in the United States. In *Health Communication. A Multicultural Perspective*. (Eds. S. B. Kar, R. Alcalay & S. Alex). Thousand Oaks-London-New Delhi: Sage Publications, Inc., pp. 45-78.

Lederman, L.C. (2010). Health Communication. The First Twenty-five Years. In J.W. Chesebro (Ed.), *A Century of Transformation. Studies in Honor of the 100th Anniversary of the Eastern Communication Association* (4th ed.), New York: Oxford University Press., pp. 236-254.

Levy, B. S. & Sidel, V. W. (2006). The Nature of Social Injustice and Its Impact on Public Health. In Social Injustice and Public Health. (Eds. B. S. Levy & V. W. Sidel). Oxford-New York: Oxford University Press., pp. 5-21.

Lie, R. & Servaes, J. (2015). Disciplines in the Field of Communication for Development and Social Change. In *Communication Theory*. 25(2015), pp. 244-258.

Lupton, D. (1994). Toward the Development of Critical Health Communication Praxis. *Health Communication*. 6(1), pp. 55-67.

Melkote, S. R. & Steeves, H.L. (2001). Communication Approach in the Modernizing of the Third World. In *Communication for Development in the Third World*. (2nd ed.). New Delhi-Thousand Oaks-London: Sage Publications,pp.103-147.

Payutto, P. A. (1998). *Sustainable Development* (Third ed.). Bangkok: Buddhatham Foundation.

Payutto, P. A. (2003). *Sustainable Development* (6th ed.). Bangkok: Komol Keemthong Foundation Press.

Payutto, P.A. (2007). *A Buddhist Solution for the Twenty-first Century* (17th ed.). Bangkok: Pimsuay Printing.

Prasad, K. (2009b). *Communication for Development. Reinventing Theory and Action, vol. 2*. Delhi: B.R. Publishing Corporation.

Sachs,W. (2013). Liberating the World from Development. *New Internationalist*. 460, March, p. 25.

Sallis, J. F., Owen, N. & Fisher, E. B. (2008). Ecological Models of Health Behavior. In *Health Behavior and Health Education. Theory, Research, and Practice*. 4th ed. (Eds. K. Glanz, B.K. Rimer, K Viswanath). San Francisco: John Wiley & Sons, Inc., pp. 465-485.

Sarafino, E. P. (2006). *Health Psychology. Biopsychosocial Interactions*. (5th ed.) N.J: John Wiley & Sons, Inc.

Schiavo, R. (2007). What is Health Communication?. In *Health Communication. From Theory to Practice*. San Francisco: Jossey-Bass, pp. 3-29.

Seidman, C., Silberg, W. M., and Patrick, K. (2013). Contemporary Issues in Scientific Communication and Public Health Education. In Contemporary Public Health (Ed. J.W. Holsinger Jr.). Kentucky: the University Press of Kentucky, pp. 171-191.

Servaes, J. & Malikhao, P. (2009). Advocacy Strategies for Health Communication. *Public Relations Review*. Doi: 10.1016/j. pubrev.2009.08.017.

Servaes, J. (2013). Introduction: Imperatives for a Sustainable Future. In *Sustainable Development and Green Communication. African and Asian Perspectives*. (Ed. J. Servaes). New York: Palgrave Macmillan, pp. 1-39.

Sorensen, K., Van den Broucke, S., Fullam, J., Doyle, G., Pelikan, J., et al. (2012). Health Literacy and Public Health: A Systematic Review and Integration of Definitions and Models. *BMC Public Health* 12:80. http://www.biomedcentral.com/1471-2458/12/80.

Spector, R. E. (2000). *Cultural Diversity in Health & Illness*. (Fifth ed.). Upper Saddle River, NJ: Prentice Hall Health.

United Nations (2008). *Achieving Sustainable Development and Promoting Development Cooperation*. New York: United Nations.

Wallington, S. F. (2014). Health Disparities Research and Practice. The Role of Language and Health Communication. In *The Routledge Handbook of Language and Health Communication*. (Eds. H. E. Hamilton & W. S. Chou). London-New York: Routledge, pp.168-183.

WHO (1946). Constitution of the World Health Organisation. International health conference; 1946, New York.

Chapter 2

HEALTH COMMUNICATION THEORIES: ME AND MY HEALTH TO PARADIGM SHIFTS

ABSTRACT

This chapter explores all health communication theories currently being used, and analyzes them in relation to development paradigms. The health communication paradigm shifts in communicating about health will be reported in this chapter. Theories in the modernization as well as the multiplicity paradigm will be analyzed and assessed. The paradigm that is recommended for its holistic approach is the multiplicity paradigm, and the reasons will be explained in this chapter.

Keywords: the modernization paradigm, the dependency paradigm, the multiplicity paradigm, Self Determination Theory (SDT), The Golden Rule of Habit Change, Social networks and social support, Community Organization and Community Building, the PRECEDE/PROCEED Model, the ecological models of health behavior

INTRODUCTION

Health communication, like health, is a discourse. The road to health status varies in accordance with the theoretical framework on which it is based.

Health communication can be understood as "the way we seek, process, and share health information" (Kreps & Thornton 1992: 2). The underlying assumption of this discourse is based on intrapersonal and interpersonal communication theories. Another way of defining health communication is "the art and technique of informing, influencing, and motivating individual, institutional, and public audiences about important health issues" (US Department of Health and Human Services [HHS] 2000). The underlying assumption of this discourse is based on the hypodermic effect of the mass media and one can see a unidirectional communication and top-down approach. The message or information is expected to intrigue the inner mechanism or efficacy of the audience. Thus, the influential mass media effects and intrapersonal communication theories are the base of this discourse. Dutta and Zoller (2008: 11-12) call the first two discourses post-positivistic and criticize them because they did not solve the structural problems in society.

McKee, Manoncourt, Chin and Carnegie (2000) present the health communication discourse as an enabling environment which incorporates socio-political-economic determinants with underlying skills in group and organizational communication (community-based participatory approach). Thompson, Dorsey, Miller and Parrot (2003) discuss health communication discourse as health, illness, and healthcare meanings being constructed, interpreted, and shared during interactions in healthcare contexts. Their underlying assumption is based on the interpretive social science. Scholars who advocate this approach to health communication consider communication as therapeutic and not separable from healthcare (Du Pre 2014: 11). Social determinants that can affect health, such as education, income, social class, and occupation, are included to understand health experiences. Textual, conversation analyses of shared meanings in health care and health context are added in the linguistic approach to health communication.

Dutta presents a culture-centered approach to health communication. The culture discourse of health communication interprets and shares the health meanings of people from different cultures (Dutta 2008: 85). The interplay of ideology, hegemony and participation are the key to understand the health behavior of the marginalized in a culture. The underlying assumption of this discourse is the critical theory and interpretive social science (Dutta & Zoller 2008: 14-15).

Each discourse of health communication mentioned above is related to a theoretical background and research framework. However, type and genre of health communication can be defined from other criteria. Babrow and Mattson (2003: 47-53) work on Craig's (1999) categorization of seven historical traditions within health communication theory. They are rhetorical, semiotic, phenomenological, cybernetic, sociopsychological, sociocultural, and critical. Here is a summary of their synthesis:

- The rhetorical tradition is about the studying of persuasive discourse and effectiveness of communication to challenge health policymakers.
- The semiotic tradition studies the intersubjectivity mediated by signs and sign systems shared among health communicators.
- The phenomenological tradition is about understanding health experiences of an individual, and the experiences of the otherness in the communication between patients and health care providers.
- The cybernetic tradition treats the health communication process as a linear information process starting from encoding, transmission, and decoding. It can as well include the feedback and the impact on the environment.
- The sociopsychological tradition of health communication is about the study of cognitive, emotional, and behavioral effects of individuals through the interactions in the socials.
- The sociocultural tradition is the study of shared new sociocultural patterns that communicating health produces.
- The critical tradition in health communication is the studying of discursive reflection of health and illness by applying the critical theory.

Apart from horizontally categorizing health communication into seven different traditions, scholars could categorize vertical approaches to health behavior and health communication. Wallington (2014: 172-174) describes these levels as individual level, group level, social/and social determinants level, system level, and community level.

Intrapersonal communication theories are, for instance, the Health Belief Model (HBM), Theory of Reasoned Action (TRA), Theory of Planned Behavior (TPB), Transtheoretical Model (TTM) or Stages of Change, and Precaution Adoption Process Model.

Interpersonal communication theories or group level theories are the Social Cognitive Theory; Social Networks, Social Support, and Health Behavior; and Stress, Coping, and Health Behavior.

Community and group communication theories are such as Community Organization and Community Building, diffusion of innovations, Theories of Organization Change.

Theories at the macro level are, for instance, the knowledge gap, agenda setting, the PRECEDE-PROCEED model, social marketing, and ecological models of health behavior.

All these categories have been developed, reviewed and promoted in the past. A new way of health communication analyses and syntheses will be explored next. Popular theories/models and research in the field of health communication will be discussed under the framework of development paradigms.

Analyzing Health Communication Theories under the Framework of Development Communication Paradigms

Communicable and non-communicable diseases are indicators of development. Poverty, income, education, occupation, ecology, and other socio-cultural factors are good determinants of the physical and mental health of an individual. Communicable diseases such as malaria, Tuberculosis (TB), HIV/AIDS, SARS, Swine flu, bird flu, etc. have more prevalence in developing countries than in developed countries. Lack of good public sanitation, poor education, lack of access to quality health care, lack of health insurance, lack of nutritious food, poor housing conditions, poor job satisfaction … induces poor physical and mental health. Non-communicable diseases such as cardiovascular diseases, diabetes, gout, cancer, asthma, etc. are caused by lifestyles and/or the interplay of lifestyle and environment. All of these can be explained by using the development paradigms used in communication for development. Rethinking health communication theories in the framework of development theories should give an insight into what needs to be done in the future.

Development and communication is depending upon each other just like a horse and a carriage. Communication, as a social process, is part of culture that passes on beliefs, worldviews, know-hows, values, experiences and so on to other generations. There will not be culture without communication! Development is a part of cultural artefacts. That is the software of the mind that induces policymakers to make structural changes. Thinking about development requires an understanding of paradigms or 'frames of meanings' or worldviews (Servaes 1999: 7). With reference to Jan Servaes' book 'Communication for Development. One world, multiple culture,' each of the three development paradigms proposed will be used as a guideline to discuss health communication theories/models and research.

The Modernization Paradigm

This paradigm is the oldest development paradigm. It emerged after the Second World War. The essence of this paradigm is that the ultimate goal of development is to become 'modern' or 'Western.' Therefore, each traditional society should improve on its economic growth and polity in order to climb up the ladder to the holy grail of living like Western people. Following the assumptions in this framework, modernization is often regarded as a synonym for Westernization (Servaes 1999: 22). Modernization bellows a path to economic success, a one-way street and an irreversible process taking off from a tradition society to modernity. That also implies a Western type of democracy. Important growth indicators used are literacy rate, urbanization rate, mass communication coverage, transportation coverage, etc.

Servaes (1999: 20-21) explains that the modernization paradigm is drawn from the philosophy of positivism, which Western scholars inherited from Aristotelian thinkers. Positivists claim that we can have positive and indisputable knowledge about certain things (Anderson 1996:6). Positivism philosophy reads that the world and the universe is deterministic (Trochim 2006). Social scientists adopted this positivist view of the world from a natural scientific epistemology, which assumes objective empiricism.

> The validity of observation; the unity of science and the singularity of explanation; the independence of theory and observation; the presence of literal meaning in both language of measurement and the language of claim; the logic of mathematics as a representation of the logic of human behavior; the incorruptibility of conventionalized methods; the primacy of prediction and the experimental method; and the necessity of generalization (Anderson 1996: 129).

Only empirical facts collected from such a scientific method can be claimed as truth; and the observer or researcher is in a neutral position from the observed so that the outcomes of research are considered unbiased. Empiricism, or quantifiable measurement and observation, is essential to the scientific endeavor and the scientific approach relies on experimentation (Trochim 2006). Statistical rules of decision are used to confer special validity to the outcomes (Anderson 1996: 131). This positivism philosophy influenced the development of sociology and psychology. Auguste Comte (1798-1857) introduced sociology in 1839. Sociology, according to Comte (Sociology 2009), is "subject to natural and invariable laws, the discovery of which is the object of investigation."

The modernization development paradigm can be drawn from Rostow's (1953) take-off model, which elaborates on the five stages of development that a traditional society takes off on the road to maturity and eventually reaches the ultimate stage of a mass consumption society. Servaes (1999: 21) reports that Rostow's stages are derived from the work of classical sociologists such as Durkheim, Toennies, the Weberian analysis of ideal models, and especially Parson's (1960) patterned variables. Not only does the modernization paradigm concern the societal level, it also concerns the psychological level of an individual. Servaes (1999: 22) observes that the development of individual needs would accelerate the modernization process.

Psychology is, therefore, closely related to modernization. Psychology originated in the mid-1800s when scientific or empiricist methods in the study of mind and behavior were introduced (about.com 2015a). Branches of disciplines in the field of psychology are diverse but two disciplines are very important to the modernization process: cognitive and social psychology. Cognitive psychology involves the study of how people acquire, process, and store information. This branch of psychology is akin to other disciplines, such as neuroscience, philosophy and linguistics (MediLexicon International 2014). Social psychology studies the feeling, behavior and thought of people, as influenced by the physical or mental image of other people. Social psychologists study social perception and social interaction as keys to understand social behavior, such as non-verbal behavior, conformity, aggression, prejudice, and leadership (MediLexicon International 2014).

Communication Perspectives in the Framework of Modernization

Let's start with *intrapersonal communication* theories. The simplest model of communication that derived from psychology is the individual response and reaction or the stimulus-response model. The main feature of the model is simply: single message→ individual receiver→reaction (McQuail 2005: 470). McGuire (1973) presented a more sophisticated version. He explains persuasion and opinion formation in a sequence of six stages: presentation, attention, comprehension, yielding, retention, and overt behavior.

According to Servaes (1999:24), the psychological or behavioral perspective on communication is related to the change of value and attitude of a person, as in the work of Rokeach (1966) and Lerner (1958). Lerner's (1958: 50) work suggests that an emphatic person has the psychological capacity to attain a higher degree of mobility, to be more future oriented, and more rational than a traditional person. According to Lerner, mobility leads to urbanization, which increases literacy, and that leads to participation in the economy and politics.

How an individual perceives and cognitively processes the information received is the core of the communication effects study or audience-centered research. The communication-effect hierarchy has three steps and each step shows linearity of knowledge, attitude, and behavior (McQuail and Windahl 1993: 190-191).

1) The learning hierarchy which postulates that the audience of a persuasive campaign is assumed to be motivated and interested, and proceeds from learning about innovation to developing favorable attitudes and to adapting of behavior.
2) The dissonance-attribution hierarchy postulates that each new behavior or experience is a stimulus to change in attitudes or affective responses, and then to learning about the preferences to cognitively support the behavior.
3) The low-involvement hierarchy developed by Krugman (1965) postulates that when an individual picks up some information of a product, tries it out (behavior) and then adjusts his/her attitude in line with the experience.

Cognitive psychology is what most of the intrapersonal communication models rely on. Other cognitivist theories in communication are the cognitive structure, cognitive response model of Fishbien and Ajzen (1975), and Olson and Mitchell (1975); theory of reasoned action of Ajzen and Fishbein (first outlined in 1970) (Anderson 1996: 203-204). Social psychology also influences some intrapersonal communication models or theories. Examples of such as theory are (1) Festinger's (1957) cognitive dissonance theory that explains how an individual adjusts to uncomfortable feelings from decisions, choices and new information received (McQuail & Windahl 1993: 29); (2) Comstock (1978)'s psychological model of television effects on individual behavior that requires empirical enquiries to study the direct effect of television viewing on the mental states, learning, and behavior of an individual (McQuail & Windahl 1993: 67); and (3) a transmission model of news learning which was modified from Comstock's model to study news recall and comprehension of the audience (McQuail & Windahl 1993: 96).

McQuail and Windahl (1993: 12-19) nicely summarize the *interpersonal communication* process that assumes linearity of sending a message from a sender to a receiver in the modernization paradigm:

> In the famous Laswell (1948)'s formula "Who says What through Which channel to Whom with What effect?" one can see the linearity and a one-way communication. The model emphasizes the effect of a message. Even though, there may be no effects at all. The context in which the communication takes place is ignored. A year later the Shannon-Weaver (1949) 'mathematical' model was invented in the Bell Telephone Laboratory in 1949. This is again assuming linearity and is a one-way process from the information source to the destination. The information source produces a message or a chain of messages. The message is formed into signals by a transmitter. The receiver reconstructs the message from the signal. A noise source is added in the communication path to be the indicator of a good message transmission. DeFleur (1966) developed the Shannon and Weaver model further to allow feedback in the communication loop. This model is no longer linear in its thinking because it presents a two-way communication between the sender and the receiver. Therefore, these models can be called transmission models (from sender to receiver).

McQuail (2005: 70) reports that the satisfaction of the audience is the measure for the efficiency or success of the message transfer. These are just a few examples of communication models that fall within the modernization paradigm.

Mass communication theories that fall within this paradigm are a communication campaign, the hypodermic needle theory, the two-step flow of communication, and the diffusion of innovations. Nowak and Waerneryd's (1985) communication campaign model is comprised of a linear flow of elements that can make a campaign successful (McQuail and Windahl 1993: 184-187). McQuail and Windahl (1993: 186) present an overview that starts from the intended effect that needs to be defined by a campaigner, to competing communication. Furthermore, the communication object (for instance, a health behavior improving object); the target population and the receiving group; the channels for different types of message and different target groups, the message which is geared toward the audience diversity; the communicator or sender who is a spokesperson of the campaign, persons as a team, or institution(s); and the obtained effect which can be intended and unintended ones, negative as well as positive. McQuail and Windahl (1993: 186) contend "the effect can be cognitive (attention and knowledge gains), affective (relating to feelings, moods, and attitudes) and conative (behavior, activity and implementation)."

The hypodermic needle theory or the bullet theory is an obvious stimulus-response model postulating that the mass media have a direct impact on the audience. The audience is passive.

Later, scholars acknowledged the fact that the audience is actually active and they are not always influenced by the mass media to change behavior. The two-step flow of communication is a correction of the hypodermic needle theory arguing that it should be a two-step of influence: first by the mass media and second by the interpersonal communication. The audience is divided into opinion leaders and followers. The opinion leaders receive ideas from the mass media and will persuade or influence attitudes and behavior of the followers during the interpersonal or group communication process (Servaes 1999: 23).

Next, the model that has been applied in many fields: the diffusion of innovations model by Rogers (and Shoemaker). Rogers is considered to be the 'father' of diffusion theory in the context of development. Rogers observed how people in agrarian societies move from a traditional life to a more technically advanced society. Rogers describes this as a linear path of adoption or rejection of the innovation process or 'diffusion.' He stresses five distinctive phases of progress towards the ultimate objective: the adoption of cultural innovation. They are awareness, interest, evaluation, trial, and adoption. Later on, Rogers and Shoemaker limited these five to four crucial steps of diffusion and adoption (Servaes 1999: 24). These four crucial steps to adopt or reject innovation are: knowledge, persuasion, decision, and confirmation. Knowledge is what a person gains when the person has awareness of the existence of the innovation; persuasion is when the individual forms a favorable or unfavorable attitude towards the innovation; confirmation is what happens when the individual seeks reinforcement for the innovation decision she/he made. That person may change the decision if exposed to conflicting messages about the innovation (McQuail & Windahl 1993: 73-74).

At a society level, Wilbur Schramm's (1964) contribution needs to be mentioned: "a developing country should give special attention to combining mass media with interpersonal communication" and mass media are the watchdogs, policymakers, and teachers for change and modernization (Servaes 1999: 25).

Health communication theories at each level of analysis will be discussed next.

Health Communication Theories vis-a-vis the Modernization Paradigm

Health communication theories that will be discussed next emerged from the field of health education and health promotion. Important theories will be analyzed. The level of analysis will be individual, interpersonal, group, and society level. Each model will be assessed and critiqued.

At the Individual Level

The Health Belief Model (HBM)

This model continues to be very popular in the health communication field. HBM emphasizes what happens in the individual beliefs system before that person takes a health action to prevent, to screen for, or to control illness conditions (all can be called 'health behavior') (Champion & Skinner 2008: 46-49). In order to act on health behavior, a person perceives the susceptibility of getting a disease or condition, first. Then, the person perceives threat of severity of an illness if leaving it untreated. The person also perceives benefits of the actions for reducing the threat from the disease or condition, and perceives barriers or negative aspects of the actions as well. Then, that person will build up self-efficacy or the conviction that s/he can successfully take the behavior action required to produce the outcomes. In other words, accept the illness or get treated.

Modifying factors of HBM are age, gender, ethnicity, personality, socioeconomic conditions, and knowledge. These factors influence all the steps before the self-efficacy is reached. HBM is used in quantitative research, such as cancer screening behavior, mammography and risk-taking sexual behavior (Champion & Skinner 2008: 53-62).

Critical Assessment of HBM

This model is positivistic; it assumes a rational consequence of events and linearity. How do we know that these phases of health beliefs happen in the same sequential fashion for everybody? For instance, the patients' point of view and the health providers' may differ and the sequence of events may differ.

This model heavily relies on quantitative data and statistical analysis. Every construct (perceived susceptibility, perceived seriousness, perceived benefits, and self-efficacy) needs to be measured. The validity of using this model is questionable as each person perceives and interprets the same construct differently. Questionnaires almost always limit the diversity of potential answers to five or so multiple choices.

Although this model considers sociopsychological variables, such as social class, peer group and reference group; demographic variables, such as race and ethnicity; and structural variables, such as knowledge about disease, prior contact with the disease, practice settings of the healthcare providers (Spector 2000: 13-16), the model fails to demonstrate how these variables influence each construct. The process from cognition to action is assumed to be linear (it may not be linear in reality, though) so that it would be possible to use inferential statistical analyses such as regression analysis. Moreover, this model assumes a static social context, which in reality is full of conflict, class struggle, and ethnocentrism. The underlying concept of power is hardly ever mentioned or taken into account.

Theory of Reasoned Action (TRA), Theory of Planned Behavior (TPB), and the Integrated Behavioral Model (IBM)

TRA postulates that an individual's beliefs about outcomes (or attributes of performing the behavior or behavioral beliefs) determines attitude, and that determines behavioral intention which, in turn, determines behavior (Montano & Kasprzyk 2008: 71). This theory is based on the assumption that the behaviors under study are under full volitional control. The theory of planned behavior adds a variable to cover the study of non-volitional control behavior: perceived behavior control. Madden, Ellen & Ajzen (1992: 5) state that the theory of planned behavior (TPB) predicts the effects of perceived control over behavior in two possible ways. First, perceived behavior control indirectly influences behavioral intention mediated by motivational factors. Second, perceived behavior control has a direct effect on behavior without being mediated by intentions. External variables that have impact on the intention to perform the behavior are demographic variables, attitude towards targets, personality traits and other individual difference variables (Montano & Kasprzyk 2008: 70).

TRA/TPB has been used in many health research settings, such as exercise, smoking and drug use, HIV/STD-prevention behaviors, mammography use, etc. (Montano & Kasprzyk 2008: 76). IBM has been used for HIV/STD prevention and condom use behavior (Montano & Kasprzyk 2008: 81). From Champion & Skinner (2008: 77), IBM is an integrated model that incorporates TRA and TPB. Three sets of phases lead to behavior. The first set of beliefs or feelings about behavior leads to attitude, then leads to intention to perform the behavior, and finally to behavior. The second set of expectations or behavior of others leads to a perceived norm, and that leads to intention to perform the behavior and to behavior. The third set of control beliefs and efficacy beliefs leads to perceived control and self-efficacy, and that leads to intention to perform the behavior and to behavior. Apart from that, four components lead directly to behavior: knowledge and skills to perform the behavior, salience of the behavior, environment constraints, and habit.

Critical Assessment on TRA, TPB, and IBM

Although TPB is complimentary to TRA in order to test both volitional and non-volitional behaviors, the model of TRA combined with TPB as IBM is still assuming linearity and has the positivist underlying assumption. It is known that attitude does not necessary lead to behavior change. Montano and Kasprzyk (2008: 81) state that other demographic characteristics such as, attitudinal and individual difference variables, and personality may be associated with behaviors.

Sequential steps of what is going on in the mind may not be the same as what is stipulated in the theory. For instance, the content of the message, the mass media, the sociocultural context have also direct effects on behavior without passing the step of perceived control or attitude. In other words, the impact of the social context or the environment, and also the ways each individual decides to act, are not linear at all. Intention to perform the behavior may come from socialization, religious beliefs, political ideology, emotion or non-rational reasons without passing through perceived control of behavior. The measurement of constructs used in the theory may not be valid because most constructs require bipolar scales and that forces the respondents of the questionnaire to rate their behavioral intention, attitude, and perceived behavioral control.

For assuming linearity in statistical analysis, the assessment of this theory is the same as that of the HBM. TRA, TPB, and IBM rely on numerical data collection for statistical analyses; close-ended questions are needed, but that is not enough to really understand other underpinning factors. Champion and Skinner (2008: 82) advise researchers to conduct open-ended questions to probe the problems more. The use of IBM for risk-taking behavior, such as condom use research, is not reliable because people will not say what they do. It has been proven by Malikhao (2007: 156, 243) that having a good attitude towards condom use, does not mean that an individual will use condoms. Furthermore, people almost always give socially acceptable answers when it comes to sex-related research.

One of the critiques of TRA, TPB, and IBM is that they are not applicable to a non-Western culture as beliefs patterns may vary across different cultures (Montano & Kasprzyk 2008: 81).

The Transtheoretical Model and Stages of Change (TTM)

"The Transtheoretical Model (TTM) uses stages of change to integrate processes and principles of change across major theories of intervention," explain Prochaska, Redding, and Evers (2008: 97). This model focuses more on changes in behavior and less on cognitive variables.

The Model consists of many constructs linked altogether in five stages of change, ten processes of change, pros and cons of changing, self-efficacy, and temptation. As explained by Prochaska, Redding & Evers (2008: 98-99), the stages of change start from pre-contemplation or no intention to take action within the next six months, until termination or no temptation to relapse and 100 percent confident about change of behavior. Each stage of change allows timing for intention to take action. Processes of change start from consciousness raising to social liberation, meaning realizing that the social norms are changing in the direction of supporting the healthy behavior change. Prochaska, Redding and Evers (2008: 103) state the critical assumptions of TTM as follows:

> "1. No single theory can account for all complexities of behavior change. A more comprehensive model is most likely to emerge from integration across major theories.
> 2. Behavior change is a process that unfolds over time through a sequence of stages.
> 3. Stages are both stable and open to change, just as chronic behavioral risk factors are stable and open to change.
> 4. The majorities of at-risk populations are not prepared for action and will not be served effectively by traditional action-oriented behavior change programs.
> 5. Specific processes and principles of change should be emphasized at specific stages to maximize efficacy."

Critical Assessment of TTM

This theory reflects the underlying modernization paradigm resembling the diffusion of innovations theory that stresses phases of change. The process of adopting a health behavior starting from awareness or consciousness raising, like a take-off phase of the diffusion of innovations, till the last stage: social liberation – realizing that the social norms are changing in the direction of supporting the health behavior change, which is like the adoption of cultural innovation of the diffusion of innovations theory. Thus, linearity still holds. The critique on statistical modeling of the above-mentioned theories still holds.

Another critique: the changing of cognitive or mental state in many stages does not guarantee the behavioral change. The intervention on any stage of change (or intentions) may not yield behavior change (Brewer & Rimer 2008: 156). A deficiency of this model is that each stage definition is pretty vague in its time frame. Brewer & Rimer (2008: 156) already assessed this time frame of stage, and concluded that it makes the measurement of stage inaccurate because of the limited recollection of the respondents.

One missing feature of this model is the sociological or contextual factor. The model assumes a static social system. It seems that social conflict and social struggles do not lead to any behavioral change in this model.

The Precaution Adoption Process Model (PAPM)

This model is a stage theory. It is different from the TTM in the sense that it refers to the psychological process within an individual, while the TTM refers to periods of time. This model assumes that people pass through different phases before they change their behaviors, just like the TTM. PAPM's stages start from the first stage, unawareness, to the second one, unengaged, to the third one, undecided, to the fourth one, decided not to act, to the fifth one, decided to act, to the sixth one, acting, and to the seventh one, maintenance (Weinstein, Sandman, & Blalock 2008: 123-145). The space interval between each stage is not equal.

Media have an influence in getting people from stage one to two, from unawareness to un-engagement by issue, and from stage two to three (from unengaged by issue to undecided about acting).

Critical Assessment of PAPM

The model assumes that people think in a series; it pays less attention to the context in which people live. The interval of stage 5, decided to act, to stage 6, acting, may not happen at all in real life, due to political, economic, and cultural constraints. Other aspects, such as linearity, paying less attention to external factors that affect the mental state, and on numerical data, are weaknesses similar to the ones assessed in the above-mentioned theories.

At the Interpersonal Level

Social Cognitive Theory (SCT) or Social Learning Theory (SLT)

This theory mediates the tension between human agency and the social structure by a new construct, "reciprocal determinism." However, SCT gives more preference to the human agency by proposing that individuals can change or build the environment. Thus, self-efficacy is emphasized. Another construct in this theory is observational learning or modeling. It contends that people can learn directly from experience, directly and vicariously from interpersonal communication and from the mass media. Learning has an impact on knowledge, attitude, and behavior.

Critical Assessment of SCT/SLT

One of the modernization paradigm characteristics one can find in SCT is the American ideology of individualism, the idea that one can thrive regardless of supporting environments or an enabling social structure. This theory pays more attention to self-efficacy but less attention to the social structure that affects knowledge, attitude or behavior. Viswanath (2008: 274) reports about one more pitfall of this theory:

> "Despite the intuitive sense that vicarious learning through media has a powerful influence on knowledge, beliefs, and behaviors, particularly in the context of so-called "entertainment-education" (or edutainment), it is difficult to test this assumption empirically using SCT without isolating other factors that influence social change and the mechanism that contribute to it."

At the Organizational/Community Level

Stage Theory of Organizational Change

This theory is based on the idea that organizations pass through a series of steps or stages as they change (Butterfoss, Kegler & Francisco 2008: 338-339). The stages start from defining problem (awareness stage), initiate action (adoption stage), implement change, and institutionalize change. The levels of changes can be at the individual level, team or work group level, and at the organizational level.

Critical Assessment of Stage Theory of Organization Change

Critiques of this theory are more or less the same as those of the theories below.

Diffusion of Innovations

This theory has been attributed to the American scholar Everett Rogers. The adoption of innovation process takes five stages as described in the beginning of this chapter. The innovations must contain certain characteristics that affect diffusion as follows: if they are considered as better than the idea, product, or program it supersedes; if they are compatible with the intended users' values, norms, beliefs, and perceived needs; if they are easy to use; if intended users can try them on; and if the benefits of an innovation are easily identified and visible to others (Oldenburg & Glanz 2008: 319-320). Adopters of innovations can be categorized in this theory as innovators, early adopters, early majority adopters, late majority adopters, and laggards. This theory assumes that when the individual adopts the innovation, that person will be an innovator or modern, no longer a laggard. This is the basic idea of modernization.

Critical Assessment of Diffusion of Innovations

The underlying assumption of this theory is ethnocentrism and endogenism. The theory is based on American settings. Exporting this theory to Third World settings has not been very successful. Diffusion of innovation theory was used in many agrarian settings in India but this theory was proven not useful. Servaes (1999: 30) explains that technology transfer from the First World to the Third World is under the control of the First World that has more power of control and uses it to serve its own interests.

Thus, this theory pays less attention to cultural differences, to environmental or socioeconomic and political factors. What happens in China regarding air pollution, cancers, communicable diseases such as SARS, swine flu, food contamination is a proof that being the innovator, and no longer a laggard, brings in so many environmental and social problems. At the same time, China's health hazards remind us that catching up with the West to reach the modernization benchmark with a primarily focus on economic growth, has brought along unwanted consequences in terms of health and environmental disasters. The diffusion theory is linear and promotes the idea of wanting to catch up with technology transfer without seeing one's own context and cultural values. Those who adopt or import technology or new ideas from somewhere will also take the values or ideas of the people who control the technology.

Social Marketing and Edutainment

These are not communication theories but "communication strategies." They are based on positivism under the modernization paradigm.

Social marketing has been used in health promotion as a strategy to bring messages across by mass media to improve on health behavior. Social marketing focuses on behavioral outcomes; gives more preference to benefits of the social than on monetary benefits; maintains an ecological perspective; develops a strategy according to the Four Ps of a marketing strategy (Product, Price, Place, and Promotion); and uses audience segmentation to gear the messages to suit the preferences of each group (Storey, Saffitz & Rimon 2008: 439).

Four health behavior theories are commonly used to guide the planning and evaluation of social marketing; they are the IBM, the extended parallel processing mode, observational (or social) learning theory, and diffusion of innovations (Storey, Saffitz & Rimon 2008: 448). All of these theories have already been discussed.

Edutainment uses the same principle as social marketing but it mixes information or education with entertainment to send health messages across to the audience (sexanddrugsandrockandhealth n.d: 3). Singhal and Rogers (1999: 9) consider edutainment as the process of purposely designing and implementing a media message to entertain and educate the audience at the same time with the purpose of altering the knowledge, attitude, and behavior to a positive level for individuals and communities.

Critical Assessment of Social Marketing and Edutainment

This strategy contains the underlying assumption of the hypodermic needle model which exaggerates the effect of mass media in changing health behavior of the audience. However, the segmentation of audiences by social marketing implies that the audience is no longer considered faceless and passive, like in the original hypodermic needle theory. Nevertheless, it remains a media- or sender-centric model, and therefore linear. Moreover, changing the behavior of the audience through strategic planning by using mass media may be successful for some audiences only. Social marketing with new media, social media for social marketing (explained in *Chapter 5*), and edutainment, if planned in concert with personal media, can be effective in awareness raising and health information publicity to encourage a change of behavior. But still, more is needed for a sustainable behavior change.

Conclusion

Health communication theories under the framework of the modernization paradigm have a tie with social psychology, social marketing, and underwent much influence from agricultural extension invented and promoted by Rogers' diffusion of innovations (Servaes & Lie 2014: 11). Extension in the 1960s, 1970s, and 1980s was the knowledge and technology transfer to help farmers in developing countries yield more crops. Dominant ideas within the subspecialty of health communication lie within the Information, Education, and Communication (IEC) and Knowledge, Attitude, and Practice (KAP); other two subspecialties are risk communication and entertainment-education or edutainment (Servaes & Lie 2014: 12, 3). Health communication in the context of communication for development concerns pandemics such as HIV/AIDS, TB and malaria, polio; new communicable diseases such as SARS, avian flu, Ebola, swine flu; and family planning and reproductive health. The public health professional as development field worker is what Kennedy (2008: 154) coins as a 'social broker,' who serves as a 'go between,' gatekeeping the flux of information between communities and groups and government decision-makers.

Dyll-Mykelbust and Zwane (2015: 65-81) studied how communication can be powerful tools to prevent Female Genital Schistosomiasis (FGS) in the Ugu district of South Africa and concluded that a top-down approach to communication was not a sustainable approach to conscientize young women to the hazardous impact the tradition could have on their health. They reported "many health interventions often lack the foresight to see that a dictatorial communication approach does not lead to sustained change in behavior" (Dyll-Mykelbust & Zwane 2015: 78). This study once again reveals that many top-down modernization approaches to health communication lack the components that would nurture sustainability. (Sustainability covers a range of quality of life improvements: human rights, equity, participation, ecological balance, and empowerment.) However, if those modernization approaches are combined with other theories from new frameworks that profess sustainability, such as social marketing and edutainment, they could become useful.

Scholars have been searching for a new development paradigm and framework. New development paradigms will be explained next.

Dependency Paradigm

Although theories derived from this paradigm do not have many applications to health communication theories as such, the critique the dependistas made about the modernization paradigm is worth listening to. This paradigm emerged in the late 1960s from neo-Marxism and structuralism, and the Latin America debate on development that lead to the establishing of the United Nations Economic Commission for Latin America (ECLA) (Servaes 1999: 31). The dependency theory posits that the world system is divided into a center and a periphery. The center or the developed country uses power to exploit the periphery or developing country with its economic and political might.

The village doctors in China, also known as barefoot doctors, were active from the 1950s until the 1980s (Bulletin of World Health Organization 2008). They are a good example of health care under the dependency paradigm. In order to remain independent from expensive Western medicine, the village doctor scheme emerged to address the local needs of medical practitioners for primary health work, such as disease prevention, primary maternal health care, education, and disease information collection. Villagers were trained for three months, six months or one year, to perform basic health work for people living in rural areas (Bulletin of the World Health Organization 2008). Acupuncture, Chinese herbal medicines, traditional healing and exercises were promoted.

This scheme later evolved under the multiplicity paradigm, as will be explained in the next section.

One of the critiques on the dependency paradigm is that it blames external sources, but pays little if any attention to the endogenous factors in developing countries. Therefore, in the

1990s, many scholars looked for a new framework, which became the multiplicity, alternative or *another development* paradigm.

MULTIPLICITY OR ALTERNATIVE PARADIGM

A report of modernization versus dependency, by Servaes (1999: 47), can be summarized as follows: The modernization paradigm is a high-tech, top-down, Americanized development model. It is unidirectional from "health professionals to receivers" assuming that the receivers are uninformed about health issues and traditional, thus, in need to be educated or upgraded through diffusion of innovation, two-step-flow, and social marketing strategies to inform about health issues; alter then attitudes toward adopting a healthy life style and health behavior change. Mass audiences were influenced by media technologies. Mass media played a major role in disseminating health, illness and disease information. Research of the diffusion approach overemphasizes quantitative criteria above social and cultural factors. The dependency paradigm, though not much used in health communication, faces more or less the same critiques as the modernization paradigm. It is a unilinear communication approach and is unidirectional: from "us to them."

Therefore, the multiplicity paradigm emerged as a viable alternative. Servaes (1999: 78-79) compiled the principles of this alternative paradigm as follows:

1) It should be based on appropriate needs of human beings, in addition to the four basic needs, on the condition that each human should be able to control their own destiny and be free from domination or exploitation.
2) Development should originate from within each society.
3) Each society should be able to rely on its own resources and strength.
4) Each society should pay attention to its eco system, natural resource management, and relevant technology.
5) Each society should realize the interdependency of resources over time (short, medium, and long term) and geo-political levels (local, national, transnational).
6) People at all levels of society should be able to partake in their governance; i.e., participative democracy.
7) Structural and sustainable changes must be implemented in a socio-economic system with the emphasis on equal distribution, and power structure change to ease self-management and participatory decision-making by stakeholders at all geo-political levels.

The multiplicity paradigm, as presented by Jan Servaes (1999), has good applications to theories, policy, and planning. It will be explicated further in this book. It is termed, 'multiplicity' paradigm because of its multidimensional development and communication model. This paradigm emphasizes interdependency between the self and the environment. Multiplicity is not based on positivism only. Rather, it uses interpretive social science to understand meanings through social interactions and the contexts in which communication takes place while adopting the more successful parts of the modernization paradigm in a mixed and matched fashion.

The modernization paradigm of cognitive reasoning tends to favor a deliberative thinking system that people are very logical, reflective, and self-controlled in the health related decisions they make. In fact it was found that people use an automatic mode of thinking most of the time; in other words, people are hard-wired to use bits and pieces of health information to reach conclusions. However, people can cooperate and build up social norms to think for the well-being of a community and attain the common good (Worldbank Group 2015: 26, 55). Thus, thinking socially as part of a sustainable development practice is more important to shift automatic thinking to social impulse.

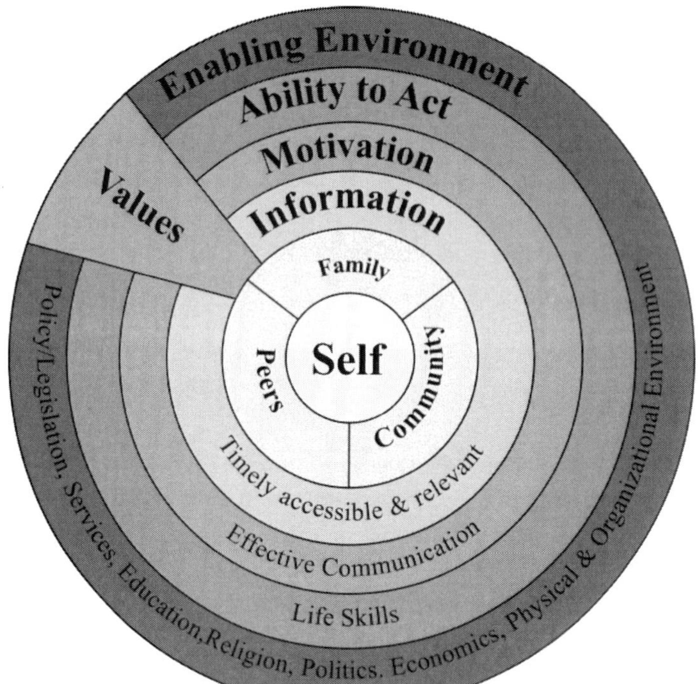

Source: Carnegie, R., McKee, N., Dick, B., Reitemeier, P. et al. (2000: 162). Making Change Possible: Creating an Enabling Environment. In (N. McKee, E. Manoncourt, S.Y. Chin, and R. Carnegie eds.) Involving People Evolving Behavior. Penang:Southbound.

Figure 2.1. The Behavior Development and Change Model.

Instead of focusing on cognitive processes, as in the modernization paradigm, the Self-Determination Theory (SDT) of Deci and Ryan (2002) is an alternative choice. Its emphasis on extrinsic motivation could be applied in this paradigm. The motivation to engage in behavioral change comes from the internalization of an individual and from the context in which that individual lives. On the individual level, a person should have first of all autonomy or the ability to control his/her own destiny. That can be achieved through empathy building and self-assessment. The person should be provided with meaningful choices in the socialization and communication process. Secondly, the environment should emphasize competency. That can be created by informal and friendly feedback on the behavior of an individual, encouragement, and understanding, instead of harsh criticism or punishment, or even rewards in the communication and socialization process. And, thirdly, that person must have a 'relatedness' with others, such as respect for others, concerns about others and positive thinking. Apart from the immediate environment of parents and family, friends, and social group members, the wider environment of culture and religion, health and education systems, news and entertainment media, influences and is influenced by our social values (Carnegie et al. 2000: 161-2, Deci & Ryan 2002: 9-20).

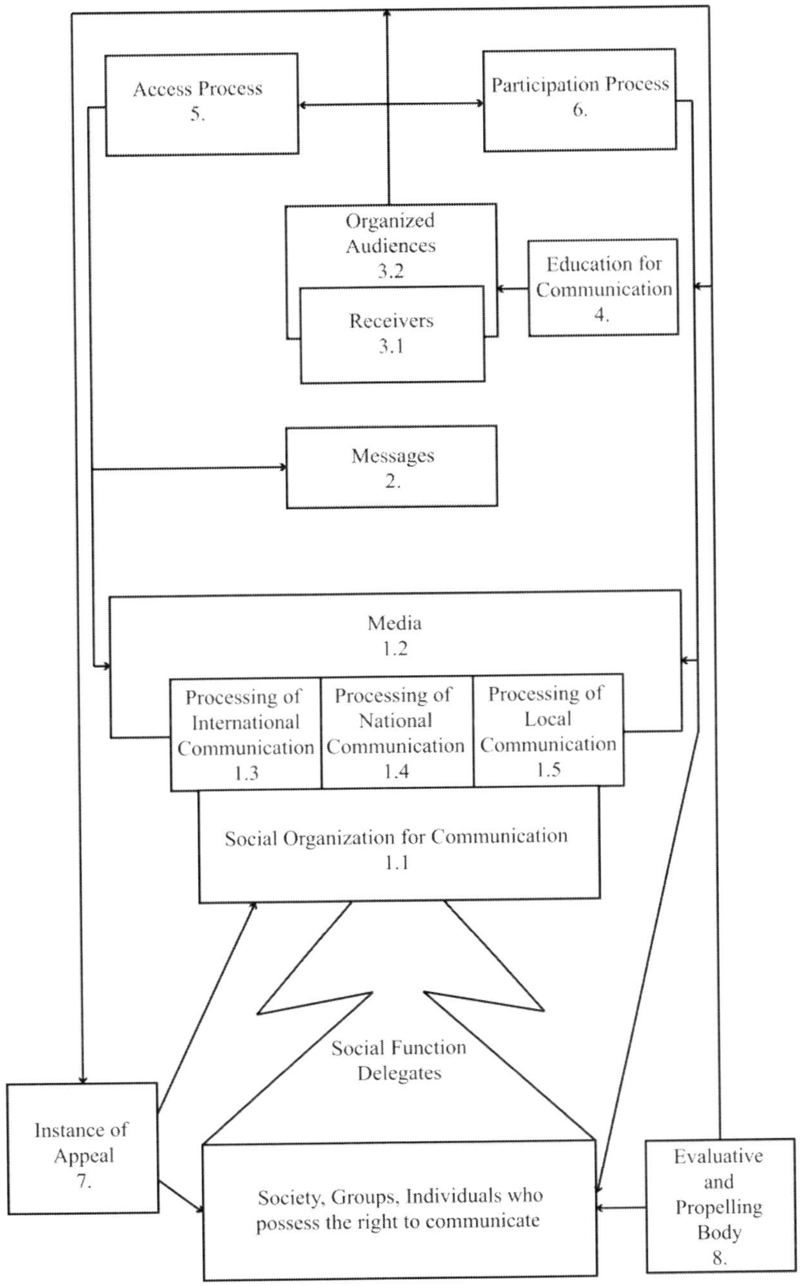

Source: Servaes, J. (1999: 90). *Communication for Development. One world, multiple culture*. Cresskill, NJ: Hampton Press.

Figure 2.2. A Communication model with active social participation.

A model proposed by Carnegie, McKee, Dick, Reitemeier et al. (2000: 157), called the Behavior Development and Change Model, is a good one for realizing all extrinsic factors that affect an individual's change of behavior.

From this model, one can see that effective communication is a fabric of social change. It leads to a community model with active social participation as presented in *Figure 2.2.*

Servaes (1999: 91) explains the elements of the model:

"1.1. Social organization for communication: the coordinating and administrative policy structure in which the media function.
1.2. Media: an organized set of transmission instruments that distribute messages under the coordination of social organization for communication.
1.3. Processes of international communication: the interrelationship between national media and the international agencies that provide messages in accordance with national and international jurisdictions.
1.4. Processes of national communication: the mechanism whereby the media and the receivers obtain a critical panorama of the national reality within the limits of their own nationally formulated norms.
1.5. Processes of local communication: the mechanisms whereby local media and interpersonal communication intermingle and contribute to local decision-making, cultural identity, participation, and so on.
2. Messages: mainly 'information' of and about events, which are received, processed, and transmitted on the basis of information for social and individual rights, previously determined at a social and global level. This information must thus provide an unfalsified, analytical treatment of the society.
3.1. Receivers: receivers of the messages, who enjoy sufficient education and adopt a critical attitude toward the message. Training should help them to become active subjects in the communication process.
3.2. Organized audiences: the receivers in their entirety. They should neither be perceived as individuals, nor as an amorphous, quantitative mass, but rather as social groups or institutions that are linked in an organizational or structural way with the society at large, such as labor unions, cultural groups, political parties, or "new social movements."
4. Education for communication: the use of educational resources at all levels of society to enable the receivers to form an opinion, to judge information, and to evaluate the role of the media as transmitters of socially interpreted events.
5. Access process: the right of the receiver to participate in the conceptualization and processing of communication and his or her potential right to use the media for further 'conscientization.'
6. Participation process: the mechanisms whereby an organized public obtains access to the structures where the internal planning and decision making about the media are done, as well as to organizations which deliver education for communication.
7. Instance of appeal: legal organisms established to support the right of the receivers to critical information and organized media participation.
8. Evaluation and propelling body: an institutional mechanism that has the object of guaranteeing the production of communication as a social right and obligation and of helping in its implementation."

Communication at all levels is important in this model as well. Communication for sustainable social change is not an isolated process; globalization, gender, social movements, and cultural diversity are incorporated in the framework to achieve four pillars of sustainability: economic viability, social responsiveness, respect for the environment, and cultural diversity (Servaes & Lie 2014: 6). This leads to the next part, communication perspectives.

Communication Perspectives in the Framework of Multiplicity Paradigm

The mode of communication, this paradigm focuses on, is not individual self-efficacy but participation of the used-to-be-called target group/audience/receivers. In this paradigm, the audience is no longer viewed as passive. Each of them is unique and can be interactive online. Participatory communication encompasses the involvement of all stakeholders; rights of everyone to engage in decision-making processes that affect their lives; accountability, transparency, corporate social responsibility, accessibility, and efficiency, as well as leadership, champions[2], and resilience[3] (Servaes & Lie 2014: 5).

Three communication levels within the framework of multiplicity paradigm can be identified: advocacy communication, participatory communication, and communication for structural and sustainable social change. *Advocacy communication* in a traditional sense means the way a representative of a social group used to convince or persuade the people in power to implement changes on the issue(s) that needs to be resolved within the community. Social advocates are issue- or program-oriented; they do not work on a continuum for the sake of community development. The social advocates assist the community at their convenience (Kennedy 2008: 156). Media advocacy means using mass media to record and present problems to the authority. A new definition of advocacy is to empower the grassroots to let their voice be heard (Servaes & Malikhao 2009: 2). Mass media can play two advocacy roles: (a) supporting development initiatives by the dissemination of messages that encourage the public to support the development project; and (b) providing the necessary information and feedback to decision-makers needed to reach a decision. Health advocacy should be viewed in conjunction with social support and empowerment strategies. This new definition is closely related to the next communication approach: participatory communication. The advocacy communication can thus be termed, "participatory-based advocacy." Both interpersonal and/or mass communication can play an important role in this approach.

Participatory communication needs capacity building, organizational skills, leadership, and commitment. The essence of the participatory model is as follows: (1) human development comes first; (2) development means empowering the local people to conserve their culture, intellect, and environment; (3) the participatory model emphasizes the local community, spirituality, diversity of culture, dialogues, and emancipation (from ethnocentrism, chauvinism, racism, nationalism, egoism, sexism, etc.); and (4) participatory development concerns a genuine and strong democratic process for strong institutions at the community level resulting in power redistribution (Servaes 1999: 93).

---

[2] Champions are the trendsetters or the flavor of the week. It combines a specific personality, behavior, knowledge, and power.

[3] Resilience refers to the ability of people to absorb, adapt, and reorganize.

Communication for structural and sustainable social change sees the development field workers (in the health communication case – health professionals) as social mobilizers who empower and encourage the community members to identify their own needs, make decisions as a group, and take action. The social mobilizer firmly believes that the social group members are capable of planning and implementing their own social change process.

Characteristics of communication for sustainable social change depend upon the following criteria:

1) Whether is it is dialectical communication, or not;
2) Whether there is participatory communication, or not;
3) Whether it allows the marginalized groups to voice their opinions, or not;
4) Whether it allows human growth, instead of material growth, or not. This includes self-reliance, – meaning that people in the community can manage their own resources in an autonomous way --, which means that the stakeholders can take their destiny in their own hands.

Health Communication Theories vis-a-vis the Multiplicity Paradigm

As reported, the health communication theories in the framework of the modernization paradigm could induce awareness and attitude change on health issues, but could rarely reach up to a level of health behavior change. Theories in the framework of the multiplicity paradigm pay more attention to the context of communication and focus on how to make the environment support the change of health behavior. This involves collaboration of multi-sectors in the society, training, leadership, capacity building, civic society, policies, planning, logistics, and health care management without losing the ground on culture, traditional health care and healing, social and economic determinants.

Health communication theory that focuses on the individual level would be the Self-Determination Theory by Ryan and Deci (2002); and at the group or organization level, the above-mentioned 'communication model for active social participation.' Carnegie et al. (2000) propose the 'Behavior Development and Change Model' to create an enabling environment for health behavior change in health projects. Some popular models, such as social marketing, social networks and social support, community organization, the PRECEED/PROCEED model, and the ecological models of health behavior, can be applied under the condition that a participatory communication model must be integrated in these models.

At the Individual Level

Self Determination Theory (SDT)

SDT sets forth that social contextual or extrinsic factors support the motivation to act of an individual. It proposes that humans have three intrinsic needs: autonomy, competence, and relatedness to others (Williams 2002: 235). Autonomy refers to the degree to which an individual is responsible and willing to perform a behavioral practice. Competence refers to a felt sense of confidence to act effectively. Relatedness concerns the extent to which an individual feels connected to others. The theory posits that the supporting or enabling social environment will enhance the psychological growth and development, and mental and physical health of an individual (Ryan & Deci 2002: 5). Williams (2002: 235) explains two types of motivated behaviors: an autonomous and a controlled one. Autonomy concerns action with a full sense of volition and choice from own interest and integrated values from others, self, and environment; whereas controlled behaviors mean to act out of pressure or seduction. This theory suggests that people will engage in behavior more autonomously when their three psychological needs are fulfilled. This involves a process called internalization, which shows how individuals develop their own self-regulatory processes from the external regulatory process (Schafer 1968). According to Williams (2002: 237), internalization has two types: introjection and integration. Introjection is a partial internalization in which regulations are being considered by people but not really accepted as their own, whereas integration means a much fuller internalization in which people consider it important and immerse its regulatory process with their own aspects of self.

Critical Assessment

This theory takes the surrounding factors into account. It gives credit to the importance of social thinking rather than automatic thinking or thinking impulsively. Communicating about health from the SDT perspective is not a linear type of thinking. A holistic approach of what constitutes health determinants, such as poverty, poor education, poor housing, poor sanitation, bad media, unsafe water and food, air quality, health policies, stereotyping, institutional discrimination, etc., needs to be taken into account. However, only survey research and laboratory experiments were conducted. More qualitative interviews should be conducted to enhance the understanding of internalization.

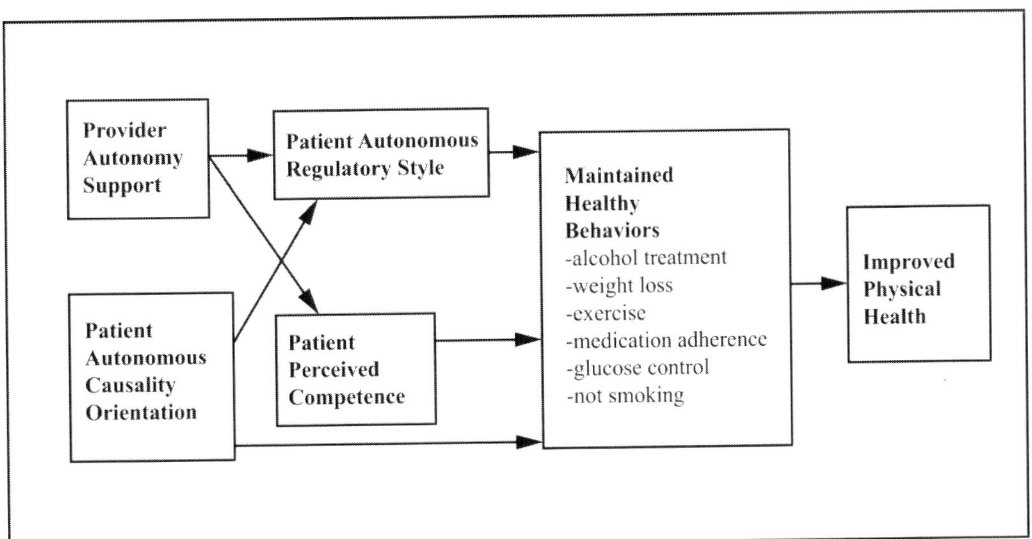

Source: Williams, G. G. (2002: 240). Improving Patient's Health Through Supporting the Autonomy of Patients and Providers. In (E. L. Deci & R. M. Ryan eds.) *Handbook of Self-Determination Research*. Rochester, NY: the University of Rochester Press, pp. 233-254.

Figure 2.3. The Self-Determination Model of Patients' Motivation Behavior, and Health.

At Interpersonal Level

The SDT can be used to explain how interpersonal communication can support the autonomy of a patient to be more responsible for his/her health behaviors. Williams (2002: 238-239) reports good research results when health care professionals or teachers take the perspectives of the patients or students into account, provide relevant information and choices, and encourage the patients' or students' health responsibility. To the contrary, controlling behavior of healthcare providers or teachers by way of rewards, punishment, and judgmental evaluation will not yield motivated health behavior.
Figure 2.3 presents both patients' and providers' conditions for long-term behavior change.

Application of the Behavior Development and Change Model in Health Communication

This model emphasizes interpersonal communication via life skill training and explicates key factors in the environment that enables the motivation and the ability of an individual to act on health behavior from behavioral pathogen[4] to behavioral immunogen[5].

Life skills are psychosocial competencies covering decision making, problem solving, critical thinking, creative thinking, communication, interpersonal relationships, self-awareness, empathy, coping with stress and emotion (Carnegie & Weisen 2000: 123). They are essential to a healthy development; they help prevent risk-taking behavior and health hazards such as drug, alcohol, and tobacco abuse, exposure to Sexually Transmitted Infections (STIs)--including HIV/AIDS, adolescent pregnancy, child abuse, injury from accidents, depression and anxiety, bullying and violence, suicidal behavior, gender and racial discrimination, school drop-out, and delinquency (Carnegie & Weisen 2000: 128). Life skills programs normally are designed for children and adolescents. However, life skill education can be geared towards specific groups: teenage parents, street children, refugee children, working youth, sex workers, unemployed youth and adults, abused women's groups, youth and adults in reform school and prison (Carnegie & Weisen 2000: 130). Intercultural communication is also required for life skill training (see *Chapter 4* for more details).

Critical Assessment

Life skills and intercultural skills are very important to communicate with subculture groups in order to reduce judgmental or stereotypical attitudes and behaviors toward the marginalized or minorities. Linker (2015: 153-168) explains that members of a community should be able to understand that the identity of a person is formed by intersectional attributes such as social class, gender, age, education, family upbringing, etc., and that they should realize the invisibility of social privilege in order to understand the marginalized. Conditional trust should be applied. This means working with as less bias or prejudice as possible and giving others more credit, emphasizing good intentions and trustworthiness. Recognizing mutual vulnerabilities is also necessary.

---

[4] Behavioral pathogen is an action that is considered to likely cause damage to health (Morrison & Bennett 2006: 61). Examples of behavioral pathogen are smoking, binge drinking, drug use, unprotected sex, eating too much transfat, etc.

[5] Behavioral immunogen is an action that is considered to be health protection (Morrison & Bennett 2006: 61). Examples of behavioral immunogen are aerobic exercise at least 30 minutes a day, wearing a seatbelt while driving, wearing a helmet while riding on a bicycle or motorcycle, eating fruits and vegetables, eating whole grain, etc.

Empathy building and compassion can be trained to reduce stress and encourage self-esteem and social acceptance; thereby, improving mental health of individuals. Empathic dialogue training should be included in the training of life skills, meaning that the members must learn the fallacies or bias in argumentation and reasoning.

At a Group/Community Level

Individuals will decide to change their behavior when s/he feels safe, supported, accepted in the community. Therefore, an enabling environment is vital. Referring to Carnegie et al. (2000: 157-211), key factors in the environment are: policy and legislation, services, education, religion, politics, economics, physical and organizational environment. A group/community involvement in health has citizen input and participation as key elements (MacLachlan 1997: 13). Let's explain:

The Golden Rule of Habit Change

Duhigg (2013: 17) reports that habits are what people do without thinking. That is a psychological process in which a part of the brain, called basal ganglia, chunks a sequence of actions into an automatic routine so that the brain can save the mental capacity for the thinking and decision making. Duhigg (2013: 19-20) explains how our brain generates a three-step habit loop. The first step: there must be a cue that triggers the brain to the second step: the routine, which can be physical, mental or emotional. And finally, when there is a reward the brain will remember. Over time, this cue and reward would reinforce each other and create a sense of anticipation for neurological craving. Eventually, a habit is born. By finding a simple and obvious cue and identifying a reward, we can create a routine, states Duhigg (2013: 36). Duhigg (2013: 34-35) explains how a toothpaste company sells their product by creating a cue of "tooth film." People are told to run their tongue across their teeth and feel "a film." Then the reward of using the toothpaste is having beautiful teeth. Millions of people are persuaded to start their daily ritual: brushing teeth with the toothpaste, which produces foam and tinkles the gum for sensational effects.

As summarized from Duhigg (2013), a habit can be a simple one like to brush your teeth, or the daily routine of how to drive to work from home. This habit will be encoded in our brain structure and rarely disappears. This is useful when we learn how to bike, swim, or drive. We will never forget the skills. Unfortunately, the brain cannot distinguish bad- from good habits. Some habits are negative health behaviors, such as cigarette smoking, binge drinking, being idle/not wanting to exercise, addicted to fast food, gambling addicting, snacking all day long, and so forth. Fortunately, there is a way to change undesirable habits: by inserting a new routine, which uses the same cue and provides a similar reward. This is how the Alcoholics Anonymous Association (AA) treats alcoholics to achieve sobriety. One thing is worth remembering: one can change the habit but one can never truly extinguish bad habits. One always needs the socials: peer pressure or a support group to help reinforce the new habit loop. By training self-discipline, choosing to build on one keystone habit or a "small win," one can change either personal or organizational habits. Will power strength is a skill that can be trained by letting the trainee write down their goals and plan each week or each day depending on which habit we want to rebuild. Teamwork, less chains of command, check and balances are crucial to change the old organizational routines. For social change, it also needs a cue and reward, but there must be strong ties or social capitals to help make the social actions ripple across the board. This leads to the next topic.

Social Networks and Social Support

Heaney and Israel (2008: 190-191) report that social networking indicates strands of relationships between individuals and socials. A person who keeps a strong social relationship is known to be healthy and to have longevity. A ramification of social networking is social support. Social support is a subset in the domain of social capital that enables social group members to health behavior practices. It supports the health behavior change in many ways: emotional, instrumental, informational, and appraisal. Emotional support concerns expression of empathy, love, trust, and caring. Instrumental support covers tangible aid and services. Information support refers to advice, suggestions, and information. Appraisal support involves information that is useful for self-evaluation.

Participatory communication can be used to enhance problem-solving processes at the community level.

Critical Assessment

Social support groups support the idea that humans are social animals. Humans need friends and contacts to feel a sense of belonging and feel accepted in a community.

People living with HIV/AIDS groups are good examples of networking to share experiences on life and treatments, and to boost up morale and mental health as well as adding an economic aspect. These groups can function as educators on HIV/AIDS prevention and reduce prejudice and discrimination within a community. Other examples can be support groups for drug and substance abuse addicts.

Community Organization and Community Building

Glanz (2008: 294-295) reports that key concepts are empowerment, critical consciousness, community capacity, social capital, issue selection, and participation and relevance. Empowerment can be used at both individual and community levels. For the individual level it is about the psychological push to motivate people to be aware of their socio-political context and to take part in social change. For the community level, it is a process to increase community competence through participation.

One goal of community building is to eradicate poverty. The fact that poverty causes declines in physical and mental health will be discussed in *Chapter 3*.

Critical Assessment

Good leadership and good health policies are not mentioned. These would make the community involvement in health leap forward. Moreover, the recognition of diversities among peoples and aiming at social justice would tie the members of a community together. Linker (2015: 50-51, 59) discusses intellectual empathy development as a way to keep the members of a community engaged in health related issues. History, power, privilege, and disadvantage of a community need to be elucidated.

The PRECEDE/PROCEED Model

This model was developed in the 1970s by Green and colleagues (1980) and was later revised to include ecological and participatory approaches (Gielen, McDonald, Gary & Bone 2008: 409). PRECEDE is an acronym for Predisposing, Reinforcing, and Enabling Constructs in Educational/Environmental Diagnosis and Evaluation; whereas PROCEED stands for Policy, Regulatory, and Organizational Constructs in Educational and Environmental Development.

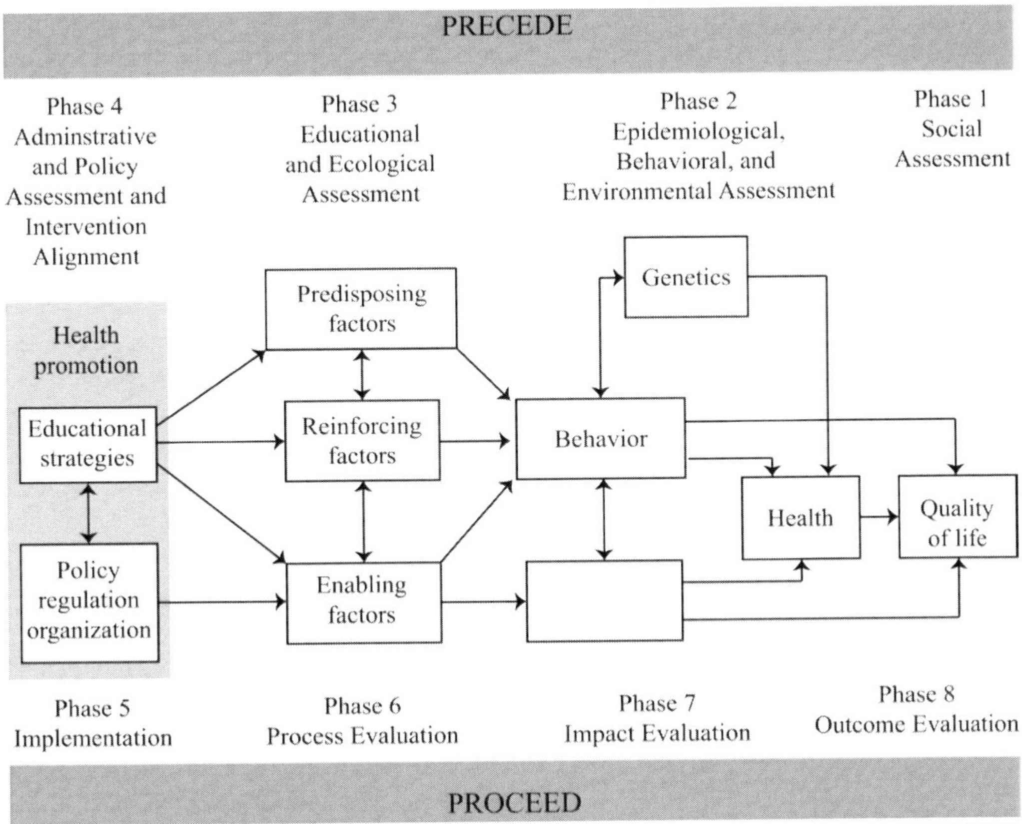

Source: Gielen, A. C., McDonald, E. M., Gary, T. L. & Bone, L. R. (2008: 410). Using the PRECEDE-PROCEED Model to Apply Health Behavior Theories. In *Health Behavior and Health Education. Theory, Research, and Practice*. (4th ed.) (Eds. K. Glanz, B. K. Rimer & K. Viswanath). San Francisco, CA: Jossey-Bass, pp. 407-433.

Figure 2.4. PRECEDE-PROCEED Planning Model.

Summarized from Gielen, McDonald, Gary & Bone (2008: 410-417), this model consists of eight phases. *Phase one* involves social assessment, participatory planning, and situation analysis. It is about gaining understanding of the community (or virtual community) by collecting multiple data from activities such as interviewing key informants, conducting focus groups with social group members, observation, and surveys. Then, assess the community needs and desires, and its problem-solving capacity, its strength and resources, and its readiness to change.

Phase two concerns epidemiological, behavioral, and environmental assessments. This includes identification of health problems, issues, or aspiration on which the program will focus. Online databases must be included. Next, three levels of behavioral determinants should be understood. First, lifestyles of the people at risk should be researched; second, behavior of others who can directly affect the people at risk; third, the action of decision makers whose decision affect the social or physical environment that affect the people at risk should be understood. Then, one needs to identify the social and physical factors or environmental determinants that can be modified to influence the health outcome or support desirable health behaviors. This second phase can make use of the Social Cognitive Theory (SCT) and organizational change theories.

Phase three concerns educational and ecological assessment. Predisposing, reinforcing and enabling factors should be identified. Change theories at individual, interpersonal and community levels can be used.

Phase four refers to administrative and policy assessment and intervention alignment. This is to identify resources, organizational impediments and facilitators, and policies useful for the implementation of programs while maintaining sustainability. This phase can use the same theories as phase three.

Phases five to eight concern implementation and evaluation.

Critical Assessment

A positive aspect about this model is that it considers rounded aspects of health determinants. It still needs leadership and empathic dialogue training in order to smooth the cooperation among community members, though. The strength and weakness of a community in health management, health services, and health literacy should be identified. The civil sector should be involved in this model. Health care volunteers and volunteers who can boost up the morale of health support groups can be a good input in this model.

However, this model overlooks the importance of the media. Instead of using the media to encourage aggression, derision, and acerbic dialogues, a project leader could use the media to create compassion and cooperation. The media can be used to teach cooperative reasoning, which is "the recognition that not all arguments have to be battles aimed at persuading and winning. Arguments about social identity and social differences should be efforts at establishing mutual respect" (Linker 2015: 96).

Participation by way of advocacy either by the mass media, online media, and interpersonal media can make or break a health project.

The Ecological Models of Health Behavior

Many ecological models were developed during the past two decades. Sallis, Owen, and Fisher (2008: 466) present four core principles of ecological models of health behavior as (1) multiple influences on specific health behavior at all policy levels; (2) influences on behaviors interacting across these different levels; (3) behavior-specific, identifying the most relevant potential influences at each level; and (4) oriented towards multi-level intervention to gain most effective in engaging behavior change.

The whole gamut of the ecological model is presented in Figure 2.5.

Critical Assessment

The Ecological Model clarifies that human health behaviors are influenced by their own culture and biosphere. This model is quite similar to the Mandala integrative model. The Mandala integrative model cannot be used as an academic research theory, but it can be useful as an aide memoire (MacLachlan 1997: 16). In the Mandala model, the life style, work, human-made environment, and sick care system are related to the personal behavior, psycho-socio economic environment, and physical environment in the community context, within a given culture and biosphere. These factors influence the mind, body, and spirit of an individual. Therefore, the well-being of an individual relies very much on the culture and physical environment in which she or he lives.

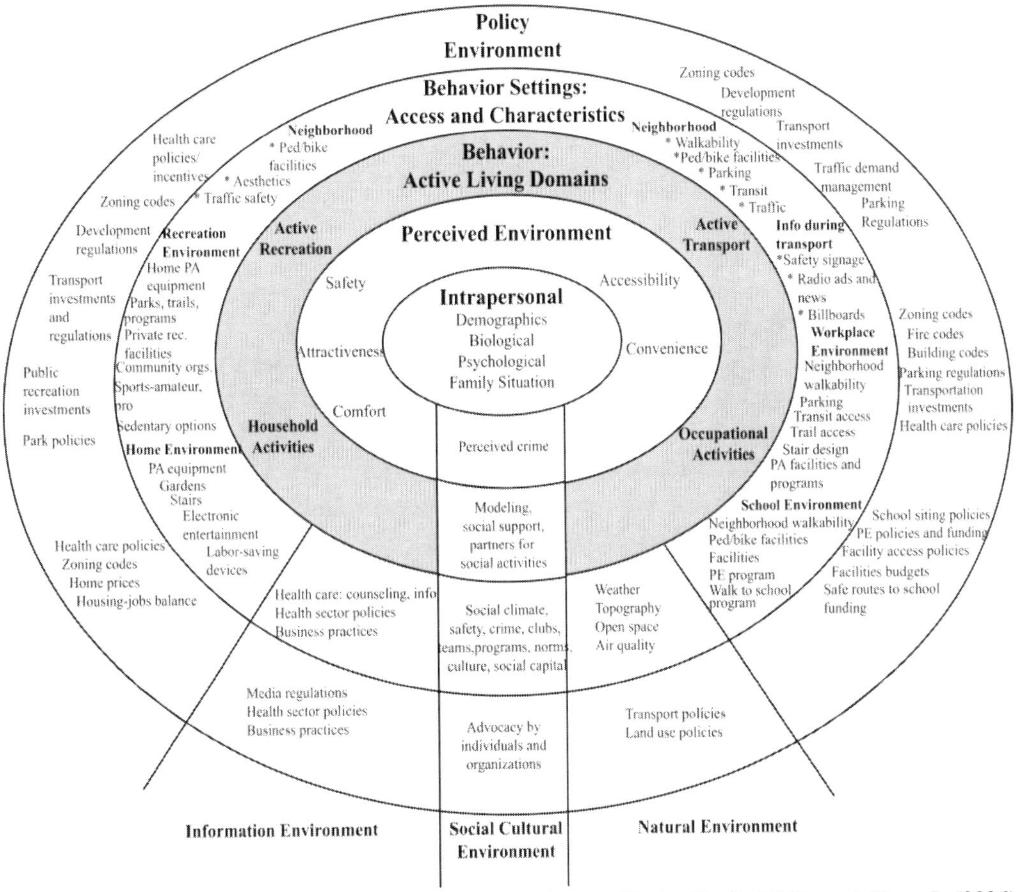

Source: Sallis, J. F., Cervero, R. B., Ascher, W., Henderson, K. A., Kraft, M.K., and Kerr, J. (2006). "An Ecological Approach to Creating More Physically Active Communities." *Annual Review of Public Health*, 27, 297-322.

Figure 2.5. Ecological Model of Four Domains of Active Living.

Good leadership, participation, and media advocacy will enhance the success of this model. At the same time the skills of dialoging and cooperative reasoning would enhance the social tie and cooperation at all levels.

CONCLUSION

This chapter has guided the reader from the modernization paradigm, which emphasizes mostly the individual's capacity and cognitive ability, growth in economic terms, and Westernization as the goal of development, to the multiplicity paradigm which views the socio-cultural context as important to encourage social thinking. Self-determination and autonomy are important for personhood development nurtured by an enabling environment at the individual level. Participation and empowerment are essential to interpersonal and community health communication in the multiplicity paradigm.

According to Janzen (2002: 79), based on a diagram in Wellin (1977: 56), McElroy and Townsend (1979: 14), Cordell, Gregory, and Piche (1992: 45-46), the ecology of health is related to institutional structures, health resources, morbidity and mortality, and demography. Institutional structures such as ideology and concepts, society and state, and food and producing technology, have an impact on health resources: water and sanitation and housing; maternal and child care, and medicine; and nutrition and access to land. The morbidity and mortality include infectious and parasitic disorders; diarrhea, gastritis entitris; influenza, pneumonia, and bronchitis; cardiovascular diseases, neoplasms, degenerative diseases, accidents and violence; and diseases of infancy. The demography includes natality (birth/1,000/year); mortality (deaths/1,000/year); and migration.

The multiplicity paradigm underpins many useful theories mentioned above. As our social identity is intersectional with so many socio-economic and cultural determinants, embracing pluralism and diversities embedded in these theories would reduce cognitive dissonance, biases, prejudice, stereotyping, and discrimination. Theories in the modernization paradigm can be selected with caution to be used under the multiplicity paradigm. Mix and match; and think globally but act locally is encouraged.

If health is a social fabric, then mass media are social lubricants. Health communication cannot be successful without thinking socially and using the media to advocate health for all. Policies and leadership are essential to close the gaps of inequality, poverty, and social injustice, which are underlying assumptions of health and well-being. That will be further explored in *Chapter 3*.

REFERENCES

Anderson, J. A. (1996). *Communication Theory. Epistemological Fou*ndations. New York-London: the Guilford Press.

Babrow, A. S. & Mattson, M. (2003). Theorizing about Health Communication. In T. L. Thompson, A. Dorsey, K. I. Miller, and R. Parrot (Eds.) *Handbook of Health Communication*. New York-London: Lawrence Erlbaum Associates, Inc., pp. 35-61.

Brewer, N. T. & Rimer, B. K. (2008). Perspectives on Health Behavior Theories that Focus on Individuals. In K. Glanz, B. K. Rimer & K. Viswanath (Eds.) *Health Behavior and Health Education. Theory, Research, and Practice*. (4th ed.) San Francisco, CA: Jossey-Bass, pp.149-165.

Butterfoss, F. D., Kegler, M. C. & Francisco, V. T. (2008). Mobilizing Organizations for Health Promotion. Theories of Organizational Change. In K. Glanz, B. K. Rimer & K. Viswanath (Eds.) *Health Behavior and Health Education. Theory, Research, and Practice*. (4th ed.) San Francisco, CA: Jossey-Bass, pp. 335-361.

Carnegie, R., McKee, N., Dick, B., Reitemeier, P. et al. (2000). Making Change Possible: Creating and Enabling Environment. In N. McKee, E. Manoncourt, C. S. Yoon, and R. Carnegie (Eds.) *Involving People Evolving Behavior*. Penang: Southbound, pp.157-211.

Carnegie, R. & Weisen, R. B. (2000). The Ability to Act: Strengthening People's Life Skills. In N. McKee, E. Manoncourt, C. S. Yoon, and R. Carnegie (Eds.) *Involving People Evolving Behavior*. Penang: Southbound, pp.121-154.

Champion, V. L. & Skinner, C. S. (2008). The Health Belief Model. In K. Glanz, B. K. Rimer & K. Viswanath (Eds.) *Health Behavior and Health Education. Theory, Research, and Practice.* (4th ed.) San Francisco, CA: Jossey-Bass, pp. 45-65.

Cordell, D. D., Gregory, J. W., & Piche, V. (1992). The Demographic Reproduction of Health and Disease: Colonial Centeral African Republic and Contemporary Burkina Faso. In S. Feierman & J. M. Janzen (Eds.) *The Social Basis of Health and Healing in Africa.* Berkeley: University of California Press.

Du Pre, A. (2014). Communicating about Health. (4th ed.) New York-Oxford: Oxford University Press.

Dutta, M. & Zoller, H. (2008). Theoretical Foundations. Interpretive, Critical, and Cultural Approaches to Health Communication. In H. M. Zoller & M. J. Dutta (Eds.) *Emerging Perspectives in Health Communication. Meaning, Culture, and Power.* New York and London: Routledge, pp. 1-27.

Dutta, M. J. (2008). *Communicating Health.* Malden MA: Polity Press.

Dyll-Myklebust, L. & Zwane, D. (2015). Uncovering Barriers to Bilharzia Prevention Communication in Ugu District, South Africa: Lessons Learned Through Participatory Communication. *Communicare. Journal for Communication Sciences in Southern Africa,* pp. 65-81.

Gielen, A. C., McDonald, E. M., Gary, T. L. & Bone, L. R. (2008). Using the PRECEDE-PROCEED Model to Apply Health Behavior Theories. In K. Glanz, B. K. Rimer & K. Viswanath (Eds.) *Health Behavior and Health Education. Theory, Research, and Practice.* (4th ed.) San Francisco, CA: Jossey-Bass, pp. 407-433.

Glanz, K. (2008). Improving Health Through Community Organization and Community Building. In K. Glanz, B. K. Rimer & K. Viswanath (Eds.) *Health Behavior and Health Education. Theory, Research, and Practice.* (4th ed.) San Francisco, CA: Jossey-Bass, pp.287-312.

Green, L.W., Kreuter, M. W., Deeds, S. G., and Partridge, K. B. (1980). *Health Education Planning: A Diagnostic Approach.* Mountain View, CA: Mayfield.

Heaney, C. A. & Israel, B. A. (2008). Social Networks and Social Support. In K. Glanz, B. K. Rimer & K. Viswanath (Eds.) *Health Behavior and Health Education. Theory, Research, and Practice.* (4th ed.) San Francisco, CA: Jossey-Bass, pp.189-210.

Kennedy, T. (2008). *Where the Rivers Meet the Sky. A Collaborative Approach to Participatory Development.* Penang: Southbound.

Kreps, G. L., & Thornton, B. C. (1992). *Health Communication: Theory & practice* (2nd ed.). Prospect Heights, IL: Waveland Press.

Lerner, D. (1958). *The Passing of Traditional Society: Modernizing the Middle East.* New York: Free Press.

Linker, M. (2015). *Intellectual Empathy. Critical Thinking for Social Justice.* University of Michigan Press: Ann Arbor.

MacLachlan, M. (1997). *Culture and Health.* Chichester-New York-Weinheim-Brisbane-Singapore-Toronto: John Wiley & Sons.

Madden, T. J., Ellen, P. S., & Ajzen, I. (1992). A Comparison of the Theory of Planned Behavior and the Theory of Reasoned Action. *Personality and Social Psychology Bulletin.* Feb. 1992 18: 3-9.

Malikhao, P. (2007). *HIV/AIDS Prevention Strategies in Two Thai Communities: Buddhist and Christian.* Ph.D. thesis. Brisbane: University of Queensland.

McElroy, A. & Townsend, P. (1979). *Medical Anthropology in Ecological Perspective*. North Scituate, MA: Duxbury Press.

McKee, N., Manoncourt, E., Yoon, C. S., & Carnegie, R. (2000*). Involving People. Evolving Behavior*. Penang: Southbound.

McQuail, D. & Windahl, S. (1993). *Communication Models for the Study of Mass Communication*. London and New York: Longman.

McQuail, D. (2005). *McQuail's Mass Communication Theory.* (5th ed.). London-Thousand Oaks-New Delhi: Sage Publications.

Montano, D. E. & Kasprzyk, D. (2008). Theory of Reasoned Action, Theory of Planned Behavior, and the Integrated Behavioral Model. In K. Glanz, B. K. Rimer & K. Viswanath (Eds.) *Health Behavior and Health Education. Theory, Research, and Practice.* (4th ed.) San Francisco, CA: Jossey-Bass, pp. 67-96.

Morrison, V. & Bennett, P. (2006). *Introduction to Health Psychology*. Harlow, Essex, England; New York: Pearson/Prentice Hall.

Oldenburg, B. & Glanz, K. (2008). Diffusion of Innovations. Montano, D. E. & Kasprzyk, D. (2008). Theory of Reasoned Action, Theory of Planned Behavior, and the Integrated Behavioral Model. In K. Glanz, B. K. Rimer & K. Viswanath (Eds.) *Health Behavior and Health Education. Theory, Research, and Practice*. (4th ed.) San Francisco, CA: Jossey-Bass, pp. 313-333.

Prochaska, J. O., Redding, C. A., & Evers, K. E. (2008). The Transtheoretical Model and Stages of Change. In K. Glanz, B. K. Rimer & K. Viswanath (Eds.) *Health Behavior and Health Education. Theory, Research, and Practice*. (4th ed.) San Francisco, CA: Jossey-Bass, pp. 97-121.

Rostow, W. W. (1953). *The Process of Economic Growth*. Oxford: Clarendon Press.

Ryan, R. M. & Deci, E. L. (2002). Overview of Self-Determination Theory: An Oganismic Dialectical Perspective. In E. L. Deci & R. M. Ryan (Eds.) *Handbook of Self-Determination Research*. Rochester, NY: the University of Rochester Press, pp.3-33.

Schafer, R. (1968). *Aspects of internalization*. New York: International Universities Press.

Servaes, J. & Lie, R. (2014). New Challenges for Communication for Sustainable Development and Social Change: a Review Essay. *Journal of Multicultural Discourses*. (http://dx.doi.org/10.1080/17447143.2014982655).

Servaes, J. & Malikhao, P. (2009). Advocacy Strategies for Health Communication. *Public Relations Review*, doi: 10.1016/j.pubrev.2009.08.017.

Servaes, J. (1999). *Communication for Development: One World, Multiple Cultures* (1st ed.). Cresskill, New Jersey: Hampton Press, Inc.

Singhal, A. & Rogers, E. M. (1999). *Entertainment-education: a communication strategy for social change*. Mahwah, NJ: Lawrence Erlbaum Associates.

Spector, R. E. (2000). *Cultural Diversity in Health & Illness*. (5th ed.) New Jersey: Prentice Hall Health.

Storey, J. D., Saffitz, G. B., Rimon, J. G. (2008). Social Marketing. In K. Glanz, B. K. Rimer & K. Viswanath (Eds.) *Health Behavior and Health Education. Theory, Research, and Practice*. (4th ed.) San Francisco, CA: Jossey-Bass, pp. 435-464.

Thompson, T. L., Dorsey, A., Miller, K. I., & Parrott, R. (2003). *Handbook of Health Communication*. (T. L. Thompson, A. Dorsey, K. I. Miller & R. Parrott Eds.) New York-London: Lawrence Erlbaum Associates.

Trochim, W. M. K. (2006). Positivism & Post-Postitivism. (http://www.socialresearch methods.net/kb/positvsm.php, accessed on April 7th, 2015).

US Department of Health and Human Services (HSS) (2000). *Healthy people 2010: Understanding and Improving Health*. Washington, DC: US Government Printing Office.

Viswanath, K. (2008). Perspectives on Models of Interpersonal Health Behavior. In K. Glanz, B. K. Rimer & K. Viswanath (Eds.) *Health Behavior and Health Education. Theory, Research, and Practice*. (4th ed.) San Francisco, CA: Jossey-Bass, pp. 271-281.

Wallington, S. F. (2014). Health Disparities Research and Practice. The Role of Language and Health Communication. In H. E. Hamilton & W. S. Chou (Eds.) *The Routledge Handbook of Language and Health Communication*. London-New York: Routledge, pp.168-183.

Weinstein, N. D., Sandman, P. M., & Blalock, S. J. (2008). The Precaution Adoption Process Model. In K. Glanz, B. K. Rimer & K. Viswanath (Eds.) *Health Behavior and Health Education. Theory, Research, and Practice* (4th ed.) San Francisco, CA: Jossey-Bass, pp. 123-147.

Wellin, E. (1977). Theoretical Orientations in Medical Anthropology. In D. Landy (Ed.) *Culture, Disease, and Healing: Studies in Medical Anthropology*. New York: Macmillan.

Williams, G. G. (2002). Improving Patient's Health Through Supporting the Autonomy of Patients and Providers. In E. L. Deci & R. M. Ryan (Eds.) *Handbook of Self-Determination Research*. Rochester, NY: the University of Rochester Press, pp. 233-254.

World Bank Group (2015). *World Development Report. Mind, Society, and Behavior*. Washington D.C: International Bank for Reconstruction and Development/ The World Bank.

Websites

About.com 2015 a http://psychology.about.com/od/historyofpsychology/a/psychistory.htm, accessed on April 9th, 2015.

Bulletin of the World Health Organization 2008 http://www.who.int/bulletin/volumes/ 86/12/08-021208/en/, accessed on June 15th, 2015.

IGI-Global 2015 http://www.igi-global.com/dictionary/positivist-epistemology/23062, accessed on April 9th, 2015).

MediLexicon International, Ltd. 2014 http://www.medicalnewstoday.com/ articles/154874. php, accessed on April 9th, 2015).

Sex and Drugs and Rock and Health n.d. http://www.sexanddrugsandrockandhealth. com/page3.htm., accessed April 16, 2015.

Sociology 2009 http://sociology-4-all.blogspot.hk/2009/03/auguste-comte-1798-1857-founding-father.html, accessed on April 9th, 2015.

Chapter 3

THE IMPACT OF GLOBALIZATION ON HEALTH AND DISEASES: IMPLICATIONS FOR HEALTH COMMUNICATION FOR SUSTAINABILITY

ABSTRACT

This chapter analyzes the impact of globalization on health and diseases. How globalization is related to uneven development in the world will be discussed. At the same time, how globalization is related to new kinds of diseases and the return of almost eradicated diseases will be assessed as well. Also Western diseases and HIV/AIDS in relation to globalization form part of this chapter. Last but not least, we discuss the impact of globalization on the environment and its relationship to health. After all, health and sustainability are interrelated.

Keywords: globalization, localization, Western diseases, HIV/AIDS, climate change, sustainability of health

INTRODUCTION

The concept of globalization must not be reserved only to phenomena in the 20th and 21st centuries. Though globalization may be a new term, historian Hopkins (2002: 1-10), sees it as a historical process from before 1500 till now. According to Lie (2003: 101-116), globalization can be understood as a flow of cultural products from one location to another. The location can be nations, communities, institutions, or individuals. Unfortunately, the global flows cannot be smooth because of nation state boundaries, geo-cultural boundaries between East and West, and geo-economic boundaries, such as the North/South divide (Powell & Steel 2011: 79). That gave birth to inequalities. Health and diseases are direct manifestations of these inequalities. To achieve sustainable development, combating inequalities are one of the major tasks of the United Nations, national and local governments and organizations, communities and civic societies. Planning for effective health communication relies on a good understanding of external factors that influence health, wellness, and diseases.

Globalization, the Irresistible Force towards Uneven Development

Globalization is multidimensional and complex; it requires diverse definitions. Definitions have some relation to concepts like modernization, Westernization, economic growth, socio-cultural and political challenges, interconnectivity of the globe, and so forth.

Many scholars state clearly that the globalization process has been an ongoing process since the archaic time. Hopkins (2002: 1-10) explains that the 'archaic globalization' period occurred from Byzantium and Tang to the renewed expansion of Islamic and Christian power after the 1500s. Hopkins then identifies the second period as 'proto-globalization,' when political and economic development became especially prominent, between about 1600 and 1800 in Europe, Asia, and parts of Africa. The third period, 'globalization,' is the colonial period from 1760 onwards. Globalization that can be related to modernity started from 1800. It refers to the rise of the nation state and the spread of industrialization. The last process, post-colonial or contemporary globalization, refers to the historical process from the 1950s till now. Hopper's (2006: 4) definition of contemporary globalization concurs. It is the process by which the world has become interconnected, and that leads to the formation of global networks, transnationalism, deterritorialization, time-space compression and the speeding up of everyday life. Held and McGrew (2007: 2-3) arrive at similar characterizations: "Globalization denotes the intensification of worldwide social relations and interactions such that distant events acquire much localized impacts and vice versa."

Globalization encompasses the reduction of barriers physically, legally, linguistically, culturally and psychologically; it makes people engage with one another without space-time barriers (Scholte 2005: 59). Scholte (2005) further reports eleven categories or manifestations of contemporary globalization: communication, travel, productions, market, finance, organizations, military, ecology, health, law and consciousness (for more details, see Scholte 2005: 49-84). In other words, globalization is about *uneven change* in form and degree in both abstract and concrete ways of the global structure and social interactions. Not everyone benefits from globalization; the winners are those who live in developed countries and the losers are mostly those who live in developing countries.

As the globalization process progresses, it is becoming clearer and clearer that inequalities exist in both degree and kind. Modernization or economic growth comes with globalization. However, globalization is not westernization, as some parts of the world are not westernized but are still modernized, such as Singapore, Taiwan and Iran (Nisbett 2003: 224). Modernization means transferring Western ideas and technological advances to Third World countries. Therefore, a new global system for transnational investments was established by a new transnational aristocracy that make countries in Latin America, Asia, and Africa become large importers of transnational goods (De Rivero 2001: 49-50). Not all parts of the world are equally modernized. In his book, "The Myth of Development," De Rivero (2001) discusses development and underdevelopment. De Rivero states that contemporary globalization is in fact "the result not so much of free global competition among nations, but of a network of agreement and productive and financial activities among the transnational corporations" (De Rivero 2001: 47).

De Rivero does not use the word "developing," because, in his view, this is just a eulogy of underdevelopment. The underdeveloped countries lack national capitalism, have huge rates of unemployment, high demographic growth, export raw material at unprofitable prices, and had no choice but to seek transnational investment (De Rivero 2001: 47). Unfortunately, transnational investments will be done in a country where the infrastructures meet the standard. Loans from the IMF and the World Bank will be the answer for developing countries. Moreover, the investors will use their power to let a developing country they choose sign agreements that allow them to benefit more (De Rivero 2001). In addition, hedge funds from transnational investors can manipulate the monetary values of poorer countries. As a result, developing countries will remain poor. Those who are rich are the G8 countries (the US, Canada, Great Britain, Australia, Germany, France, Italy, and Russia). China is rising in its GDP to become an economic giant in the world but the level of inequality and uneven development remains high. Development in China has been at social costs and costs of environmental degradation and poor health. China is a case in point to show the negative side of modernization (Malikhao 2013a).

Lee (2003) states that globalization involves three dimensions: spatial, temporal, and cognitive. The *spatial* dimension concerns the altering force of globalization to physical or territorial space, and the reconfiguration of social space towards trans-border or non-territorial relations (Lee 2003: 62, 64). This involves migration of humans, transporting animals and plants across borders, information flow, cash flow, goods and services across national borders. This also includes the negative sides of globalization, such as human trafficking, drug trafficking, money laundering, and global climate change (Lee 2004). New social spaces emerged, such as the virtual reality and cyberspace, to substitute the old notion of "global village," which means "a community in which people are connected by computers, television, etc. and all depend on one another" (Merriam-Webster 2016). It is worth noting that people in this interconnected world may not share the same taste or the same lifestyle. Rather, they tend to adopt and modify the information received via information and communication technologies and the World Wide Web to suit their lifestyle and culture. That is called *localization* (Thompson 1995, Lie 2003).

Next, the *temporal* dimension is about how we perceive and experience time. Time is being crunched as the social interactions around the world have becoming accelerated (Lee 2003: 106). This involves multi-tasking and at the same time our lives are slowed down by information overload and the complexity of organizational systems (Lee 2004).

Lastly, the *cognitive* dimension is about how globalization affects how we think: in terms of transnational corporation, the deregulation and privatization in the global economy, research and policy in the global industry, trade in cultural goods[6] or cultural products, a globalization discourse which influences public policy and opinion, and information and communication gaps between the rich and the poor (Lee 2003: 137).

In sum, globalization affects how we see ourselves and the world and what is being catalyzed by the new media: the social media and the Internet. The other main change agents are the mass media, the advertising industry, consultancy firms, research institutions, political

[6] They are print media enterprises, radio and television companies, news and features agencies, advertising and public relations firms, syndicates and independent companies producing and distributing print, visual and recorded material for print and broadcasting conglomerates, public or private information offices, data banks, software production, manufactures of technological equipment and so on. Productions from the communication industry are also known as the cultural industry because they record and reproduce cornucopia of social interactions, representations and organization systems in diverse media forms such as books, arts, films, recordings, television, radio, the internet, plays, concerts and music (MacBride 1980: 96-97). Since, also ICTs, the Internet and digital and online social media could be added to the list.

parties, religious groups, etc., and that affects our wants or perceived needs, values, beliefs, knowledge and aspirations (Lee 2004).

Without the mass media as weaving threads in the globalization process, the differences between the global and the local would not have been prominent. Martin and Nakayama (2004: 6) describe five aspects of the influence of communication technology on cultures: an increase of general information about the citizens of the world and the cultures; increased contact with peoples who possess "the otherness"; increased contact with people within the same culture for support; redefine one's own identity and think of identity management; and the gap of access to communication technology, or the so-called digital divide. These aspects together with the changing in immigration patterns and demographics result in a culturally diverse society across the globe. The mass media (and communication in general) help define and redefine local cultures and identities by helping create a global consciousness, by which people can compare how others live within their own locality via the mass media (Nash 2000: 53). Most often mass media diffuse their messages globally but the consumers of the mass media consume the messages locally, the process of which is called *the axis of globalized diffusion and localized appropriation* (Thompson 1995).

Impacts of globalization on different aspects of cultural identification, such as occupation, gender, race, religion, sexuality, sense of community, and so forth are what concerns many scholars; for instance Chen & Starosta (2004: 11), Cohen (2006: 165), Nisbett (2003: 224), Holmberg (1998: 1-17), or Featherstone (1996: 60).

THE IMPACT OF GLOBALIZATION ON HEALTH

Globalization makes some regions become centers of economic growth while other regions are outliers or closer to the periphery. Past Human Development Reports of the United Nations Development Program (UNDP) reveal that the richest one-fifth of the world population consumes 86 percent of all the world's goods and services, while the poorest one-fifth consumes just 1.3 percent. There is some evidence that the income gap between Western Europe and Africa has become 10 times wider within a decennium (Sernau 2014: 62). The gap within nations has become wider as well. South Africa, countries in Latin America and Eastern European countries have been reported to be the world's most unequal countries (Sernau 2014: 63). During the past couple of decades, the US has become the number one country of inequality among wealthy advanced nations (Sernau 2014: 64). From the aforementioned evidence, centers and peripheries occur among nations and within nations. That affects the life of the people in those regions a great deal. Harris and Seid (2004: 16) explain that the transition from agrarian to industrial societies in most developing countries has been slower and more problematic than in the developed nations, as there are many people who did not benefit from these developments. Non-communicable diseases or NCD (i.e., cardiovascular diseases, especially coronary heart disease and stroke, cancer, chronic respiratory disease, and diabetes) kill about 36 million of the world population each year (WHO 2015 a). Social determinants, that can be considered negative consequences of globalization that can contribute to NCD among populations, include i.e., the migration of the population from their traditional means of subsistence, urbanization without provision of standard housing and employment, the large unregulated marketing of tobacco products and alcoholic beverages

(Harris & Seid 2004: 16, Yach & Beaglehole 2004: 214-215). The globalized world equipped with high speed transportation means, mobility, and migration has been deemed responsible for the emergence of new patterns of infectious diseases, and has speeded up the transmission rate of the diseases. Major infectious diseases have killed large populations: small pox (killed 500 million people), measles (200 million), Spanish flu (80 million), Bubonic plague (75 million), AIDS (40 million), and typhus (4 million) (Anitei 2007). Although the incidence of infectious diseases dropped from 40 percent to 17.5 percent between 1990 and 2010, new diseases have emerged at the rate of one or more per year since the 1970s. According to the Levin Institute of the State University of New York website (2014), several new infectious diseases are, for instance, the severe acute respiratory associated coronavirus (SARS-CoV), henipaviruses (Hendra and Nipah), avian influenza virus, the H1N1 virus (swine influenza), and – the latest – Zika virus. There are also historic infectious diseases that are re-emerging again, such as West Nile fever, human monkey pox, dengue, tuberculosis, and malaria.

Uneven growth or socio-economic disparities/differentials/gaps between the haves and the have-nots posed by globalization as a threat to healthy individuals or communities can be studied in nine different approaches, according to Wermuth's research (2003: 9-43):

First, the *'health gradient' descriptive model*, which linearizes the socioeconomic status (or SES) and health outcomes, can be used to (partially) explain that high level of income, education, and occupation have some association with lower death rate (Anderson & Armstead 1995: 213-215). To elaborate, low income people and paupers face a short life expectancy from birth as they have less access to appropriate health care, nutrition, hygienic living conditions, and later in life they are more prone to chronic stress because of unstable job or unemployment prospects.

Second, being healthy or not is a consequence of *biopsychosocial effects* (Anderson & Armstead 1995: 213-225). The socio-demographic (i.e., age, ethnicity, gender, and location) together with the socioeconomic status (SES) (i.e., education, income, occupation, family wealth, perceived SES, economic mobility childhood SES, material possessions, trading/bartering practices, and national income distribution); the social environmental and medical (i.e., residential characteristics, occupational environment, social support, social/professional hierarchy, and access to health care), the psychological and behavioral (i.e., psychological distress, personality factors, health promoting behaviors, and health damaging behaviors), and physiological (cardiovascular, immune, muscular, endocrine, height, and weight) determine health and illness of a person.

Third, a paradigm for research on *SES and Health* by Williams (1990: 81-99) is based on the second approach but emphasizes more the psychosocial factors that have an impact on health: health practices (smoking, alcohol, nutrition); social ties or social support; perceptions of control; stress (family, occupational, and residential).

Fourth, the general theoretical model of *relationships between occupational quality and poor physical health* of Wickrama, Lorenz, Conger & Elder (1997: 363-375) emphasizes the underlying occupational quality, social integration and marital integration to sense of control of an individual which leads to health-risk behaviors and poor physical health.

Fifth, Kennedy, Kawachi and Prothrow-Stith (1996) found that the *degree of income inequality correlates with mortality rates and infant mortality.*

Sixth, the *social capital*, which is comprised of community cohesion and trust, a person possesses was suggested to be a good indicator of health by Kawachi and Kennedy (1997).

Seventh, the model *Social, Psychological, and Physical Pathways to Health Outcomes,* developed by Brunner and Marmot (1990: 20), reveals that social structure, social environment, and work affect the psychological aspect of an individual. This is inter-related with the health behaviors of that person. The brain of that individual subsequently creates neuroendocrine and immune responses that cause pathophysiological changes which consequently affect organ impairment and health in general.

Eighth, Wilkinson (1997) stated that improvements of the *standard of living and quality of life* via globalization lower the rate of communicable or infectious diseases, but increase the rate of non-communicable diseases, such as cardio vascular diseases, among both the upper and lower social classes.

Ninth, the *political economy* not only consists of global political and economic forces, the state, government, social classes, public administration, policy making, and the distribution of sources between and among populations, but also concerns a transnational trading system and the mobilization of labor and resources to maximize profits. In turn, it affects the living conditions of workers and their health.

Globalization is linked to health in four different layers of the socials: individual lifestyle factors, social and community influences, living and working conditions, and general socioeconomic, cultural, and environmental conditions (Lee 2005: 14). Global changes could affect health in many ways. First, patterns of population mobility could affect the genetic makeup of populations and cause certain genetically inherited disorders. Second, via global marketing and advertising industry, new patterns of consumption and lifestyle emerge as a result of the change of cultural values and beliefs. That causes lifestyle diseases, also known as non-communicable diseases, such as obesity, cardiovascular diseases, diabetes, respiratory diseases and cancer. Third, social policies imposed and enacted across countries affect access to health care. Fourth, the world economy growth leads to the employment of workers without appropriate health and safety protection measures. Fifth, the socioeconomic inequality gaps within and across many countries give rise to poverty and poor health among certain population groups (Lee 2005: 14).

Contemporary globalization is the result of a network agreement and productive and financial activities among the transnational corporations (de Rivero 2001: 47). Developing countries need to seek transnational investment as they lack national capitals; resulting in huge rates of unemployment, high demographic growth, and raw material exports at unprofitable prices. De Rivero (2001: 59-71) explains that indirectly, through the IMF joined by the WTO and World Bank, – which de Rivero called the supranational clergy as they subdued all developing countries to the *Washington Consensus* --, social inequalities have been increased more because the technological advancement in these countries cannot compete with the developed countries, and the excessive protection of intellectual property exercised by developed countries makes the copy and adoption of foreign technology to develop their own practically impossible. Within developing countries, inequalities exist because levels of urbanization differ overall. Big cities account for larger Gross National Products (GNP) than rural areas. Urbanization happening at a fast speed often results in ghettos or slums, environmental degradation, poor healthcare services, and other basic service capacity issues such as lack of water supply, proper sanitation, and waste disposal management. Urban poverty is a consequence of urbanization for those who do not benefit from the growth and opportunities globalization brings.

Poverty is directly related to ill health as it leads to poor nutrition, crowded housing and a decaying environment, poor quality medication, poor health services, poor mental health, and poor education. Moore, Gould, and Keary (2003: 271) report a list of 37 primary and secondary health indicators developed from data collected in 62 countries:

> "The eleven primary indicators included infant, child, and maternal mortality rates; incidence of malaria, measles, gastro-intestinal illness; percentage of children wasted, stunted, and percentage of wasted adult females. Secondary indicators included gender-specific infant and child mortality and life expectancy, immunization rates, various indicators related to HIV, tetanus incidence, cholera incidence, use patterns of oral rehydration therapy, and rates of availability of hospital beds and physicians."

High rates of infant mortality and low rates of life expectancy can be observed in most poor nations. HIV/AIDS, Tuberculosis and Malaria are more prevalent in developing countries than developed countries. The change of lifestyles, norms and values, leads to overconsumption and that causes environmental destruction and health hazards.

Lee (2004) reports that the spatial dimension of globalization can affect health risks as mobility of people around the globe helps spread communicable diseases such as HIV/AIDS, Tuberculosis, Malaria, Severe Acute Respiratory Syndrome (SARS), plague, etc. The mobility of unhealthy people from middle- and low-income countries to high-income countries has been a concern for rich countries. On the other hand, rich countries can pose health risks to poorer countries by exporting unhealthy products such as tobacco and fast food (Lee 2004). However, the brain drain of qualified health professionals from developing countries to developed countries is also the result of globalization. The temporal dimension of globalization has a direct impact on health. Via modern transportation systems, disease outbreaks can happen around the world. But, at the same time, modern technology allows the health communities to manage health risks faster. Last, the cognitive changes brought by the cultural goods industry that makes people need and imitate the Western lifestyle internationally or the urban lifestyle domestically has facilitated global non-communicable or lifestyle diseases. At the same time, a global consciousness of ethical values and standards of health care systems have been formalized in health policies around the world as well.

Globalization and New Diseases, and Resurgence of Nearly Eradicated Diseases

Infectious diseases that are spreading in the contemporary globalization period are many, such as HIV/AIDS, Tuberculosis, Malaria, Ebola virus disease, etc. Some diseases have been eradicated thanks to vaccination campaigns, such as Smallpox in 1977 in Somalia, and Rinderpest (which is a disease that affected livestock); some diseases are on the verge of eradication, such as lymphatic filariasis (Elephantiasis), polio, measles, mumps, rubella, and pork tapeworm (The College of Physicians of Philadelphia 2015). However, emerging diseases, defined by the World Health Organization (2016) as "one that appeared in a population for the first time, or that may have existed previously but is rapidly increasing in incidence or geographic range," are partly due to globalization. They are antimicrobial resistance, avian influenza, cholera, influenza, and chikungunya. Antimicrobial resistance is caused by many bacteria that changed their DNAs to become antibiotic-resistant. According to WHO (2015 b) five percent of patients worldwide have multi-drug resistant TB and the cost of treating this new form of TB is very expensive; in the US and in the European Union, around 23,000 and 25,000 deaths occur annually because of antibiotic-resistant infections.

New disease outbreaks emerge each year. Most of the time, they become epidemics or pandemics due to the mobility of postmodern people and communication/transportation technology. The outbreak of the Middle East Respiratory Syndrome (MERS) is a good example. It was first reported in Saudi Arabia in 2012 and since has spread to many countries, including the US. It became an epidemic when it emerged in the Republic of Korea in May 2015 (CDC 2015). Interestingly, some new emerging diseases are diseases once found in animals only. Avian Influenza or bird flu is a case in point. It is a relatively new disease discovered for the first time in 2013 in China (CDC 2014 a). This was good evidence that animals can transmit viruses to humans, such as happened after the swine flu (H1N1) in 2009, and mad cow disease turned pandemic during 1996-2006 respectively. What we learned from the swine flu epidemic is that virus from birds and swine can merge with the human flu virus and develop itself into new kinds. It resulted into new problems not related to the human seasonal H1N1 viruses that were discovered since 1977 (CDC 2010). In 1988, England and Ireland experienced the outbreak of the mad cow disease or Bovine Spongiform Encephalopathy (BSE), and later in 2003 the US detected this disease (CDC 2015). This disease causes a deterioration of the central nervous system from unknown reasons;[7] it is transmissible among adult cattle due to human's feeding the animals with parts of brains and spinal cords of the diseased ones to reduce the production cost (WebMD 2013). About eight years after the first outbreak, in 1996, the disease developed itself to infect human in a form known as Variant Creutzfeldt-Jakob Disease (vCJD). People who ate beef from infected animals developed similar symptoms as the infected cattle (WebMD 2015 a).

WESTERN DISEASES AND GLOBALIZATION

Interestingly, diseases that once thought nearly eradicated have resurged in both developed and developing countries. These are, for instance, diphtheria, scarlet fever, whooping cough, measles, and polio-like diseases that caused partial paralysis in children in Australia and the US (PBS 2014). Taking a closer look, it was found that global migration is the cause. The explanation is that unvaccinated travelers returned to their community with declining immunity and brought back a nearly eradicated virus (PBS 2014). From the globalization period in 1800s to the contemporary globalization period, starting in 1950s till now, people have migrated across borders and continents more and more. Migration has many causes. Wars, political unrests, famines, and human right abuses make people move in search of a better life. Many of these people are economic migrants. Moving from one environment to another needs adjustment of one's lifestyle, values, norms, etiquettes, or in sum, culture, to suit that of the host country. This has impacts on both physical and mental health. According to Pollard (2008), migrants who changed their dietary pattern and lifestyle

[7] An expert in nutrition suggested that feeding cattle with grains instead of grass may have affected the immunity of the cattle. Naturally cattle eat grass. In the contemporary globalization period, cattle are fed with grains such as corn (which is mostly genetically modified in the US to resist pests and insects) to reduce production costs. In the long run, this may have affected the protein of the cattle (Campbell & Campbell 2006).

have a higher chance to get the so-called Western diseases due to the adaptation of genes. Not only are the migrants to the Western world linked to Western diseases, more affluent people in the centers of the Third World or developing world get Western diseases as well as urbanization and economic development grows and people consume the lifestyle of Western people.

Western diseases like coronary heart diseases, type 2 diabetes, colon-, and breast cancer are known as lifestyle diseases or diseases of affluence. Western diseases are non-communicable diseases that were found among the top 10 causes of death in high-income countries (North America, Western Europe, Australia and New Zealand) in 2012. Those top 10 causes of death are ischaemic heart disease, stroke, trachea bronchus, Alzheimer disease, chronic obstructive pulmonary disease (COPD), lower respiratory infections, colon rectum cancers, diabetes mellitus, hypertensive heart disease, and breast cancer (WHO 2015 c). All of the afore-mentioned diseases are non-communicable diseases but some are not considered Western diseases, such as respiratory diseases. The real cause of Western diseases are the change in diets over many years from high fibers (from fruits and vegetables)/grains, low fat, low sodium and sugar to low fiber, high (saturated –either from animal or from palm oil) fat, trans-fat (from hydrogenated vegetable oil), high sodium and high sugar and refined carbohydrates (Nestle 2013: 7-17, 77, 315-334; Ruiz-Nunez, Pruimboom, Dijck-Brouwer, et al. 2013). To elaborate, the globalization of the food industry, together with the free market economy, and advertisements and the change of lifestyle patterns from slow to fast life, have altered the dietary patterns of the population in the high- income countries from slow food or self-prepared food to fast food; from fresh foods to pre-cooked, cooked, frozen and canned foods; from a few choices of soft drinks and alcoholic drinks to many choices, etc. Apart from too much salt and sugar diets that cause hypertension and metabolic disorders, the sedentary lifestyle, meaning lack of movement as a result of white-collar jobs and lack of sufficient aerobic[8] exercise, cannot help burn enough calories gained from a high calorie diets intake. Other factors are lack of sleep, chronic stress, and pollution (Ruiz-Nunez, Pruimboom, Dijck-Brouwer, et al. 2013).

Ruinz-Nunez, Pruimboom, Dijck-Brouwer et al. (2013) delved into why Western lifestyle has caused Western diseases. To elaborate, over the course of human evolution, humans' brains are larger than other animals and that has made humans extremely sensitive to glucose deficits. Humans had faced long periods of adaptation during, for instance, starvation, pregnancy, and infection/inflammation, became insulin[9] resistant to spare glucose for feeding the brain, to feed the infant during the third trimester of pregnancy, and to activate the immune system. Fatty acids in the body help repair the insulin resistant tissues during infection and inflammation by redirecting cholesterols to the damaged area. This is how the immune system is related to the metabolic system. Western lifestyle triggers a state of chronic systemic low grade inflammation which leads to the chronic compensation of the state of insulin resistance that leads to greater risk of metabolic syndromes such as diabetes mellitus, hypertension, high cholesterol, heart disease, breast cancer, etc. Determinants that may cause

[8] Aerobic (or cardio) exercises mean a kind of exercise that make the heart pump oxygenated blood to deliver oxygen to all muscles; example of aerobic exercises can be simple such as walking, jogging, hiking, dancing, running or using cardio machines, taking a yoga or aerobic class, cross country skiing, and kick boxing (MedicineNet.com 2015). The best result should be a work out for at least 30 minutes a day.

[9] Insulin is a hormone produced by the pancreas that makes our body's cells take up glucose from the blood. Insulin regulates how the body uses and stores glucose and fat (Endocrineweb 2015).

chronic systemic low grade inflammation, which Ruinz-Nunez, Pruimboom, Dijck-Brouwer et al. (2013) adapted from Egger and Dixon (2011: 339-345), are listed below:

Lifestyle

Lifestyle factors concern diet, exercise, and nutrition which, in the long run, can disturb the biochemistry balance in our body. Postmodern people have a different lifestyle than their forefathers. They are more sedentary. They socialize more, meaning eating larger portions, or more frequently, and drink sugary drinks and alcohol. Nestle (2007: 8) reports a survey result that, on average, Americans in 1996 ate 2,000 calories compared to 1,800 calories in 1970s. They consume more high-fat diets; they eat more chemicals or non-food products put in processed foods such as chemicals that give food a longer shelf-life, or enhance the flavor or texture of food. Also the food industry uses hormones, antibiotics, pesticides, insecticides, and genetically modified products in the process of producing meat, poultry, eggs, dairy products, and agricultural products for human consumption. Moreover, pollution in the sea makes seafood risky to eat for fear of heavy metals and toxins.

1. Lack of Exercise

The use of modern transport systems, private cars, and desk jobs prevents people from burning excess calories in daily life. The excess calories would be converted into adipose or fat tissues which may be distributed internally or under the skin. Adipose tissue has endocrine and immune functions that could promote inflammation and increase the risk of cardiovascular diseases, type 2 diabetes, and the metabolic syndrome (Summerfield 2012: 5, 141).

2. Nutrition

We are what we eat and what we eat could bring in free radicals, excessive fat, excessive sugar and salts, and toxins into our system. Here below is a list of what we take too much or too little of and that causes imbalances in our body.

a. Excessive Alcohol Consumption

Alcohol is causally related to major health consequences. Barrie (2012: 21-22) reports that alcohol is causally related to tuberculosis, diabetes, liver diseases, heart diseases, etc. It is also partly attributable to many sorts of cancers (mouth, pharynx, esophageal, etc.), hypertensive heart diseases, etc. Heavy alcohol consumption impacts on cancer, liver cirrhosis, and strokes.

b. Excessive Energy Intake

This comes from consumption of energy-dense foods in excessive amounts. The food industry provides highly processed foods that are high in fat and calories. Consuming lots of refined carbohydrates, meat products, soft drinks, and alcohol provides the body with excessive fuels that need to be burnt during exercise. If not burnt, it will be stored as fat tissues in the body.

c. Starvation

Famine and poverty cause starvation. Also eating disorders such as Anorexia Nervosa and Bulimia Nervosa result in emaciated or underweight bodies. This is an issue of self-image. Servaes and Malikhao (2011: 67- 69) report globalization has a profound impact on the individual level, in such a way that a person pays more attention to his/her physical appearance than before as s/he stays connected 24/7 on social media platforms. Selfie pictures, plastic surgery, losing weight to imitate photo models or movie stars are symbolic representations of this new kind of individualism in the contemporary globalization period. This new kind of individualism was already observed by Elliot and Lemert in 2006 as a highly risk-taking, experimenting and self-expressing individual underpinned by new forms of apprehension, anguish, and anxiety. In 2007, James reported about "affluenza" that causes depression and anxiety (will be explained later). Twenge and Campbell (2009) report about the narcissism epidemic, resulting in a very positive and inflated view of self.

Fairburn (2008: Table 11.2) reports that starvation (by any means) and eating disorders affect the person in psychological, behavioral, social, and physical ways. Psychological effects can result in inflexible thinking and mood swings. Also, behavior and social changes are noticeable, such as obsessiveness and lack of spontaneity, hoarding objects, and self-focused. Last but not least, physical effects result in a weaker heart, decline in sex hormone production, and deterioration of bone strength.

d. Consumption of Fast Food or Western Style Diet

As stated in the beginning of this chapter, globalization has caused not only centers and peripheries in the world, it also caused centers and peripheries within a nation state. People in the centers of developing countries imitate the lifestyles of people in the developed countries, as shown via the mass media through global marketing and advertising. Nestle (2006: 64) reports that a lot of money is spent to advertise and market soft drinks, candy bars, breakfast cereals, potato chips, and fast food in general, but little goes to promote fresh fruit and vegetables.

A Western style diet, also known as the diet of the industrialized world, is rich in fat, salt and sugar, but with low fibers. That includes high glycemic indexed (GI[10]) foods and drinks such as refined carbohydrates, sugary and artificially sweetened drinks, etc., and high animal proteins. All of these will be explained next.

A high-fat diet concerns saturated fats and/or trans-fatty acids. Food that contains high saturated fat is whole milk, whole milk products like cheese and butter, animal fat, and certain fat from plants such as palm oil. The dairy industry stimulates milk production by treating cows with a growth hormone, known as bovine samatotropin (bST), which is genetically engineered. Moreover, when a cow produces more milk, she needs antibiotics as her udders have a greater chance to become infected (Nestle 2006: 69).

Margarine was produced to substitute butter and was advertised as healthier than butter. In 1975, it was found that margarine, which contains partially hydrogenated vegetable oil (which is also used to produce shortening, crackers, snack foods, and baked goods to give them a longer shelf-life), introduces trans-fat from its hydrogenation process. Trans-fat raise

[10] The glycemic Index (GI) ranks the carbohydrate-content of foods and drinks, measuring how fast they release glucose in the blood stream that makes blood sugar levels rise (Bee 2013: 16).

blood cholesterol levels and the risk of heart disease (Nestle 2006: 110-112, Summerfield 2012: 171).

Summerfield (2012: 181) and Nestle (2006: 140) report eating too much meat (not exceeding 35% of total calories or 1.6 g/kg body weight) creates two health problems. First, proteins from meat above the level that our body uses to maintain tissue, and for other physiological functions, will be disassembled and eliminated by the kidneys. That may cause kidney damage in the long run. Another health problem is that meat of any kind is high in saturated fat. Eating meat increases blood cholesterol levels and is responsible for heart disease, cancer, diabetes, autoimmune disease, and disease of the kidneys, bones, eyes, and brain. Further than that, cheap food that includes genetically modified corns and grains, instead of grass, or even mixing ground parts of dead animals or non-food, artificial hormone and antibiotics in the process of meat production, pose health risks to consumers, not to mention that many meat industries avoid their responsibility to clean-up pollution caused by chemical fertilizers and fuels that run the machinery (Nestle 2006: 140).

Eating fish (both finfish and shellfish) seems to be a good solution, but all fish in the contemporary globalization period contains polychlorinated biphenyls (PCBs) (Nestle 2006: 204). The United States Environmental Protection Agency (US EPA 2013) explains that PCBs are man-made organic chemicals used in hundreds of industrial and commercial applications such as transformers and capacitors, plastics, fluorescent light ballasts, etc. They have been found all over the world because of their mobility in air, water, and soil and they do not break down even though they were banned in 1979. PCBs have been proven to cause cancer and to affect immune, reproductive, nervous, and endocrine systems (US EPA 2013). Another toxin found in fish is methylmercury, which is toxic for pregnant women as it can go to harm the brain and nervous system of the fetus (Nestle 2006: 188). Methylmercury is caused by falling mercury from coal-burning power plants in waterways; microorganisms in the water mythylate it and convert it to methylmercury (Nestle 2006: 187). These aforementioned facts counter the fact that fish, like salmon or tuna, contain omega-3 fatty acids that can reduce the risk of sudden death and coronary heart diseases. Thus, good advice is to eat only two servings of fish a week (Nestle 2006: 183-184).

Due to rush hours and hectic work, people in the industrialized world consume less fiber from fresh fruits and vegetables, even though it is known that plant-based diets provide relatively low calories but are high in vitamins, minerals, fiber, and other phytochemicals of plants that are good for health (Nestle 2007: 6). Dietary fiber comes from plant cell walls which are comprised of non-digestible carbohydrate and lignin; the soluble part is linked to reduce blood cholesterol; and the insoluble part helps speed the getting rid of toxins and waste materials through the colon (Summerfield 2012: 158). The reason why people in the industrialized world eat less fiber is only partly the choice of the individuals. The marketing of the food industry, advertising companies for the food industry, and food politics make it convenient for consumers to buy prepared food, prepackaged food, frozen food, canned food, snacks, etc. However, those foods are made sweet, fat, and salty in the form of "added value" to fresh fruits and vegetables. In a competitive food marketplace, consumers are encouraged to eat more. Food portions in restaurants are larger to keep the production cost low (Nestle 2006: 17-21, Cardello & Garr 2010: 13-21).

When it comes to sugary foods and sugar-sweetened drinks and artificial sweeteners, consumption of sweetened carbonated beverages and forms of candy provide low nutritional values. Excessive sugar consumption causes obesity as sugar will be converted to glycogen and stored in muscles and liver. In the globalized world, high-fructose corn syrup, dextrose, molasses, fruit juice concentrates, etc. are in the production of processed foods and snacks – in sum, they are sugar. High-fructose corn syrup has been identified as the culprit for Western diseases (Summerfield 2012: 161). Sugar, as well as carbohydrate provides four kcal of energy per gram of weight. Refined carbohydrates in processed foods, such as cakes, pastries, pasta, pies, crackers, pretzels, etc., provide more calories than whole grain carbohydrates (Nestle 2006: 310). Consumers of processed and fresh food need to consider the GI and the glycemic loads (GL[11]) of the foods.

Lastly, salt is another culprit. Eating too much salt increases the risk of high blood pressure and, therefore, heart disease and stroke. Unfortunately, salt is used in the food industry for processed foods and junk foods. One of the reasons is that salt functions as a preservative.

3. Obesity

Obesity is a state of the body mass index (BMI[12]) higher than 30. It is linked to Western diseases and high rates of depression (PsychCentral 2015). It is influenced by genes as well as eating and exercising patterns, and other individual and social factors (Schneider 2006: 270).

4. Weight Gain

Weight gain is the result of physical inactivity and the consumption of more calories than our body needs. It is a health impair. It is related to obesity.

5. Smoking

Research indicates there is also a clear link between lung cancer and smoking. The Framingham Study has tracked citizens of Framingham in Massachusetts for five decades and reports high blood pressure, high blood cholesterol, and smoking as risk factors for heart disease and obstructive pulmonary diseases (Schneider 2006: 67, 495).

6. Unhealthy Lifestyle

Lifestyle is not only an individual choice but also influenced by the environment in which people live. Urbanization as a result of economic development has some negative impacts on health in terms of crowded housing, air pollution, noise pollution, poor sanitation, and hazards from pollutions, or occupational exposure to health hazards, exploitation and sexploitation. Poverty is partly responsible for unhealthy lifestyles: injuries are twice as high in low-income areas compared to high-income areas; also the poor tend to risk having house-fires, pedestrian fatalities, and homicides more often (Schneider 2006: 294).

7. Stress/Anxiety/Depression/Burn out

Wilkinson and Pickett (2009: 42) explain how inequalities caused by globalization have psychosocial impacts on the people in developed and developing countries differently. For those living in a developed country, they lose their sense of individual identity in the crowd of the mass society; they are vulnerable to pursue their identity through consumption and that

[11] How much we eat of GI foods can have a huge impact on our blood sugar level; that is called the glycaemic load or GL (Nestle 2006: 315).

[12] BMI is a measure of body fat based on height and weight. BMI = weight (kg)/[height (m)]^2 (CDC 2015).

causes anxiety. Moreover, competition causes stress and burn out. For those living in the developing world, poverty causes anxiety, stress, and depression; the poor have a precarious life, and are constantly living under uncertainty (Agyeman 2013: 24-25). Poor people lack opportunities to physical activities and that can increase stress, anxiety, and depression. Last but not least, people suffer from "affluenza," (James 2007), a disease of wanting more material possessions to keep up appearances, fueled by the media and the interconnectedness in the contemporary globalization period. A person can be envious if s/he does not have enough to keep up with the Joneses and that can result in depression and anxiety among millions. This happens in both developed and developing worlds.

8. Sleep Deprivation

This can be caused from working long hours or trading sleep for more work or play, or the stress of daily life. In the short term it reduces performance and alertness; causes memory and cognitive impairment; stresses relationships; causes poor quality of life, occupational injury, and automobile injury (WebMD 2015 b). In the long run it causes high blood pressure, heart attack, heart failure, stroke, obesity, psychiatric problems, including depression and other mood disorders, Attention Deficit Disorder (ADD), mental impairment, fatal and childhood growth retardation, injury from accidents, disruption of bed partner's sleep quality, and poor quality of life (WebMD 2015b).

9. Age

Schneider (2006: 495) reports that, as people get older, the behaviors that most significantly affect their health are smoking, obesity, and physical inactivity. See more in *Chapter 4*.

10. Environment

a. Low Socioeconomic Status

Socioeconomic status consists of educational attainment, income, and occupation. Low socioeconomic status puts people at risks of chronic diseases. Yach (2006: 260) reports that those who are less educated tend to die from tobacco-related diseases. In developed countries, obesity can be found among those at low socioeconomic levels, regardless of race or ethnicity (Summerfield 2012: 10). Marmot and Bell (2006: 35) explain that the obesity rate among women with low socioeconomic status is higher than that among men, because higher-status women can better maintain their body weight with stronger cognitive control for diet and exercise. Summerfield (2012: 10) explains why people with low socioeconomic status are facing health risks as many socioeconomically disadvantaged communities in the US have limited access to fresh and lower-fat foods. People do not necessarily receive low-fat or low-calorie foods donated foods from community agencies. People may not know how to cook healthy food or lack the equipment to cook it. They may not be able to pay for membership to a fitness club. They may live in an unsafe neighborhood which restricts their outdoor activities. Finally, they may have less access to quality health care and regular check-ups with healthcare professionals.

b. Perceived Organizational Injustice

Yach and Beaglehole (2004: 224) report urbanization without adequate employment is a cause of an unhealthy lifestyle. The unemployed and the underemployed are not able to maintain good dietary intake, for a healthy lifestyle. They often engage in a range of substance abuse and unhealthy behaviors. Food, alcohol, and tobacco companies spend billions of dollars promoting unhealthy behaviors to young generations.

Yach (2006: 266-268) reports that in high-income and certain middle-income countries, chronic diseases are caused by life time exposure to social class, ethnicity, and gender inequalities. In the US, racial injustice contributes to chronic diseases as it was found that hypertension, HIV, diabetes mellitus, and trauma were prevalent among blacks. Risk factors for chronic diseases in developing countries have increased due to low health literacy levels, limited access to health messages, and exposure to global marketing of tobacco, alcohol, and salty, sugary, and fatty foods, the lack of coverage of government information on healthy diets and behavior to the poor communities. Tobacco products, alcohol and unhealthy foods have been targeted toward specific subgroups such as young people, ethnic minorities, and low-income populations. To make it worse, poor people in developing countries lack long-term health care services and access to quality health care.

c. Indoor and Outdoor Air Pollution

Air pollution is a result of industrialization and urbanization. The emission of exhaust fumes from cars, factories, and coal-based power plants in the environment becomes a health hazard. Indoor air pollution is not only caused by cooking, heating, and lighting, but also natural sources such as radon and chemical pollutants from building materials and cleaning products. Air pollution increases the risk for respiratory and heart diseases, and cancer (IARC, WHO 2013).

d. Second-Hand Smoking

It is also known that environmental tobacco smoke, which is a mixture of smoke from the lighted cigarette, pipe, or cigar (also known as sidestream smoke) and the smoke exhaled by a smoker (also known as mainstream smoke), has been linked to heart disease and cancer (American Cancer Society 2015).

e. Sick Building Syndrome

This is a kind of acute sickness or discomfort from spending time in an office building. It is typically marked by headaches and respiratory problems, which can be caused by poor ventilation, poor building design, occupant activities, or airborne contaminants (EPA 1991).

f. Atmospheric Carbon Dioxide (CO_2)

Carbon dioxide is the main component in the exhausting fumes or emissive smoke stacks in the environment. It is the culprit of global warming as it creates the greenhouse effect.

GLOBALIZATION AND HIV/AIDS

Not only are non-communicative diseases, especially Western diseases, caused by globalization, communicable diseases such as HIV/AIDS and respiratory diseases spread wide and far so that they become epidemic or pandemic due to the speedy real-time connection with air travel. Globalization has led to an increase in worldwide mobility of people: migration and migrant labor, tourism, displacement, occupying military forces and rapid urbanization (Lee & Zwi 2003: 18).

HIV/AIDS is a manifestation of underdevelopment. It is a social problem as well as a biomedical problem. It is a complex consequence of gender inequality; sexuality and culture; poverty; migration; urbanization, drugs and alcohol control, public health policy; capacity building among civil servants, the civic society, the mass media and the new media, and the stake holders as well as capacity building at the international levels; the (sex) education system, the public health system, and the grassroots. Globalization in this case concerns the localization of sexual practices, norms from the West, prevention strategies from the public health sector down to the grassroots level, the global prevention strategies from the UN agencies down to developing countries. This includes the bilateral or multi-lateral cooperation for support, control, and prevention (see Malikhao 2007, 2012 for more details).

HIV emerged for the first time in a developed country among men who had sex with men in 1981 in the US (Lee & Zwi 2003: 14), but later on it spread among heterosexuals more in developing countries. It is interesting to see that HIV prevalence in developed countries is controlled quite effectively, but it is more prevalent in developing countries due to many factors. As explained in the beginning of this chapter, those who are still catching up with the process of globalization are less able to adapt engaging in HIV risk-taking behaviors, and have less access to HIV counseling and testing, safer sex education, and antiretroviral drugs. Poverty in many developing countries forces people to sell unscreened blood for a living which caused the spread of HIV during the first decade of the outbreak of HIV in the 1980s. Later blood screening improved in certain developing countries, including China. The HIV epidemic in China concerns three different sociocultural and economic factors. First factor is a complex consequence of the poorly controlled blood trade, the drug trade and the sex trade. Second factor is at the cost of three socially marginalized populations: impoverished rural residents in central China, ethnic minorities in border regions, and female migrant workers in many cities. The third factor is homosexuality among Chinese male (Jun & Worth 2010:13-41).

Another factor is the sharing of unsterilized needles among intravenous drug users/ prisoners. It has been one of the causes of the spread of HIV in the developing world. An illegal witch-doctor who provides a tattooing service while using an unsterilized needle or a sterilized needle with many customers out of poverty and ignorance also causes the spread of HIV. Malnutrition and untreated venereal diseases also increased chances of HIV infection. In addition, migration spreads the HIV virus. Young migrant workers from poor countries have more chances to end in the sex trade. For some cultures, having many sexual partners is tolerated for males, while at the same time condom use as a safer sex practice is not fully implemented/enforced. The reason is not the cost of a condom, but, in some cases, the condom stands as a symbol of mistrust in an intimate relationship. Another reason is religious, as certain sects of Christianity and Catholicism prohibit condom use. The globalization of sexuality as a consequence of the mass media consumption has become another reason why HIV still persists and is more prevalent among younger generations (Malikhao 2013). The HIV/AIDS epidemic is a case in point to show that there is a relationship between the global economy, political power, AIDS epidemiology, the impact of global telecommunications and the mass media. Therefore, the impact of globalization on health should be high on any policy agenda (Lee & Zwi 2003: 30-31).

GLOBALIZATION, CLIMATE CHANGE AND HEALTH

Globalization is a threat to the environment due to the further acceleration of industrialization, transportation, and international trading. These man-made effects on the climate result in global warming due to greenhouse gas emission; the ozone depletion in the stratosphere above the Antarctica; an imbalanced ecosystem; desertification; and all sorts of chemical pollution (Harris & Seid 2004: 35). To elaborate, indicators of global warming are the rise of the temperature around the globe that affects the melting of icebergs in the North Pole and influences the rising of the sea levels; the flowering of the trees sooner; the shifted range of seasons; increase intensity of tropical storms; and salt-water intrusion into fresh water supplies (NASA 2015, Harris & Seid 2004: 36). The greenhouse gasses, which trap heat in the atmosphere and cause global warming, are emitted from industrial processes, agriculture and livestock, as well as household activities. Carbon dioxide, methane, nitrous oxide, and fluorinated gases are highly important in global warming (EPA 2015). The website of the National Geographic (2015) reveals that ozone depletion has been caused by the emission of chlorofluorocarbons (CFCs) which are found mainly in spray aerosols used by industrialized nations for much of the past 50 years. When they reach the upper atmosphere called stratosphere, where ozone layer functions as a natural belt to shield the earth from the harmful ultraviolet B from the sun, the chemicals will be broken down by the ultraviolet B-rays into substances that comprise chlorine. Next, chlorine reacts with ozone and destroys massive ozone molecules that filter the ultraviolet B radiation to the earth.

Transportation and international trading cause changes within the biodiversity of the planet, resulting in the simplification of the ecosystems, the dispersal of species between previously unconnected ecosystems, the extinction of some species, and the genetic erosion of others (Perrings 2014: 479). The latter problem concerns a hybridization of certain species due to natural cross breeding or human induced crossbreeding.

Health Effects of Global Climate Change

The depletion of ozone allows the ultraviolet B to reach the earth directly and cause skin cancer and cataracts in humans and animals. Moreover, the ultraviolet B reduces the phytoplankton populations that are food for fish and sea (National Geographic 2015). Harris and Seid (2004: 34-37) report that global climate change brings about many invasive species proliferated by global climate change and the breakdown of natural ecosystem breed water-borne diseases and diarrhea organisms; cause worldwide reduction of cereal grain production due to depleting fresh water supply; increase vector-borne diseases such as malaria and dengue fever, yellow fever and several kinds of encephalitis. Hong (2000: 68-72) added more environmental impacts on health: overfishing and depletion of fish stocks cause the loss of main protein sources; suffering of people from land scarcity due to soil erosion, salination, water logging and chemicalization; exposure to endocrine disrupting synthetic pollutants in the environment cause male and female reproductive disorders, neurological toxicity, low birth rates, and slowed fetal development; increasing lead emission, mostly in the Third World, are retarding the development of children's brains and their IQ levels; chemicals used in farming and food industry cause salmonella and listeria epidemics; the transfer of antibiotic resistance from livestock and poultry to humans, and new diseases in animals that can transfer to humans; and the loss of food, medicines, energy, and fibers as a result of biodiversity loss.

Conclusion: Towards the Sustainability of Health

To achieve sustainability of health, one must acknowledge that health and well-being has to be addressed at the individual, the social, the environment, and the global level. All levels are interacting with one another and that affects an individual's health.

Sustainability of health should mean the reduction of inequalities that affect health at all levels. We should start from the assumption that every individual should have a right to good health. This means that the peoples – rich or poor; male or female or the third gender; black or yellow or white, or mixed; old or young, no matter where they live – should have the rights to non-toxic food, clean air, clean water, good and affordable healthcare and services, and a decent society where people put "us" before "me," where racial and gender discrimination is monitored and under control. People should be taught about the carbon footprints they will leave from birth to death. Sustainability has to go along with rights, justice, and sufficiency. An individual's health and well-being will not be achieved if the environment is polluting and the society we live in is unsafe, and there is no space for humanity.

Rights imply democratic participation of all stakeholders and redistribution of resources to reduce inequalities. Rights go along with accountability and responsibility. Sufficiency implies using natural resources in moderation, redefining needs and wants, and being at peace with the ecosystem. This needs the implementation at a global, national and local level by way of agreements, laws and the protection to ensure the justice of land use, food safety, non-toxic seas and waterways, re-education, etc. Rights and justice have to go together. This needs to be learned in a good education system.

Sufficiency also means cultivating self-contentment through education. A sufficient economy emphasizes the reduction of our carbon footprint. Re-educate people to be aware that the identity of a person does not depend on how much he or she consumes should be the first and foremost agenda. So far we can see that the global politico-economy, culture, environment, social justice, food industry, medicine industry, healthcare system and healthcare services, energy industry, transportation, mobility, the mass media and the new media, are accounting for our health. Our choice of lifestyle is determined by our education, career, income, gender, social class, socialization, motivation, and self-control. All of these can be considered under the theme of sufficiency, rights, and justice.

Raworth (2012: 4) explains in a model he constructed that the sustainability of health is not a stand-alone attribute.

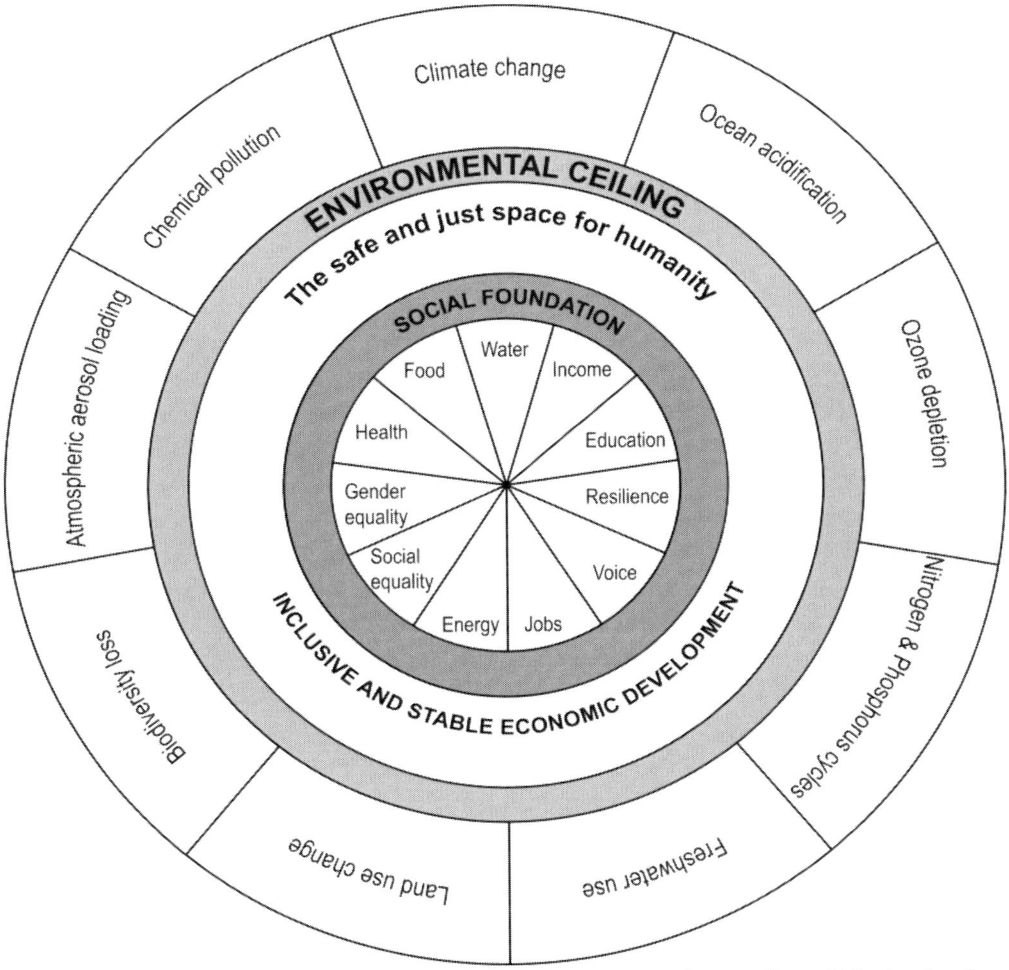

Source: Raworth, K. (2012). A Safe and Just Space for Humanity. Can we live within the doughnut? Oxfam Discussion Papers, p. 4 https://www.oxfam.org/sites/www.oxfam.org/files/dp-a-safe-and-just-space-for-humanity-130212-en.pdf, accessed January 20th, 2016.

Figure 3.1. A safe and just space for humanity to thrive in: A first illustration.

I would like to read and interpret this model as follows: the environmental ceiling is determined by chemical pollution, climate change, ocean acidification, ozone depletion, nitrogen and phosphorus cycles, fresh water use, land use change, and biodiversity loss. That needs an inclusive or participatory democratic and stable economic development that ensures the safe and just space for humanity to establish a social foundation. To achieve a good social foundation, health can be seen as part of sustainability among the rights and justice for food safety, water safety, sufficient income, good education (meaning cultivating moral ethics, humanity, environmental concerns, sufficient concepts, and cultural sensitivity as well as knowledge in arts, science, world history, world geography and technology), resilience to live in harmony with nature, rights to voice justice and equity, jobs without being exploited, social equity, and gender equality. I would like to add rights to a just healthcare system and rights to be informed about food, medicine, and anything else that impacts our health and well-being.

The right to be informed is a way to achieve social equality. That is related to the essence of this book: effective communication to attain health sustainability.

In this chapter, understanding how globalization affects health is an open door to understand the complexity of socio-political and economic determinants on individual's health. Inequalities in a sociological and anthropological perspective will be presented and discussed in the next chapter.

REFERENCES

Agyeman, J. (2013). Introducing Just Sustainabilities. Policy, Planning, and Practice. London-New York: Zed Books.

Anderson, N. B. & Armstead, C. A. (1995). Toward Understanding the Association of Socio-economic Status and Health: A New Challenge for the Biophychosocial approach. Psychosomatic Medicine 57(1995): 213-225.

Anitei, S. (2007). Top 10 Infectious Diseases That Have Killed Millions of People. (http://news.softpedia.com/news/Top-10-Infectious-Diseases-That-Have-Killed-Most-People-70741.shtml, accessed on January 29th, 2016).

Barrie, K. (2012). Alcohol. Policy and Practice in Health and Social Care. Edinburgh, Scotland: Dunedin Academic Press Ltd.

Bee, P. (2013). The Food Swap Diet. London: Piatkus.

Brunner, E. & Marmot, M. (1999). Social Organization Stress, and Health. In M. Marmot & R. G. Wilkinson (Eds.), Social Determinants of Health. Oxford, U.K: Oxford University Press, pp. 17-43.

Cardello H. & Garr, D. (2010). Stuffed. An Insider's Look at Who's (Really) Making America Fat and How the Food Industry Can Fix It. New York: Ecco (an Imprint of Harper Collins Publishers).

Chen, G.-M. & Starosta, W. J. (2004). "Communication among Cultural Diversities." In G.M. Chen & W. J. Starosta (Eds.) Dialogue among Diversities. Washington D.C: National Communication Association, pp. 3-15.

Cohen, D. (2006). Globalization and Its Enemies (J. B. Baker, Trans.) Cambridge, MA: Massachusetts Institute of Technology Press.

De Rivero, O. (2001). The Myth of Development. London and New York: Zed Books.

Dolinoy, D. C. (2015). Early-Life Exposures and the Epigenome: Interactions between Nutrients and the Environment. In E. Ho & F. Domann (Eds.) Nutrition and Epigenetics, pp. 3-52.

Dyll-Myklebust, L. & Zwane, D. (2015). Uncovering Barriers to Bilharzia Prevention Communication in Ugu District, South Africa: Lessons Learned Through Participatory Communication. Communicare. Journal for Communication Sciences in Southern Africa, pp. 65-81.

Egger, G. & Dixon, J. (2011). Non-nutrient Causes of Low-grade, Systemic inflammation: Support for a 'Canary in the Mineshaft' View of Obesity in Chronic Disease. Obes Rev, 12(5), pp. 339-345.

Fairburn, C. G. (2008). Cognitive Behavior Therapy and Eating Disorders. New York: Guilford Press. (http://www.wales.nhs.uk/sitesplus/866/opendoc/225354, accessed on September 8th, 2015).

Featherstone, M. (1996). Localism, Globalism, and Cultural Identity. In R. Wilson & W. Dissanayake (Eds.) Global Local: Cultural Productions and the Transnational Imaginary Durham and London: Duke University Press., pp. 46-77.

Harris, R. L. & Seid, M. J. (2004). Globalization and Health in the New Millennium. In R. L. Harris & M. Seid (Eds.) Globalization and Health. Leiden & Boston: Brill, pp. 1-46.

Held, D. & McGrew, A. (2007). Globalization/Anti-globalization. Cambridge-Malden MA: Polity Press.

Holmberg, C. B. (1998). Sexualities and Popular Culture. Sage Publications: Thousand Oaks.

Hong, E. (2000). Globalization and the Impact on Health. A Third World View. Document prepared for the People's Health Assembly, December 4-8, Savar, Bangladesh.

Hopkins, A. G. (2002). Introduction: Globalization – An Agenda for Historians. In A. G. Hopkins (Ed.), Globalization in World History (pp. 1-10). London: Pimlico.

Hopper, P. (2006). Living with Globalization Oxford. New York: Berg. (http://search.ebscohost.com/login.aspx?direct=true&db=aph&AN=20921322&site=ehost-live, accessed on June 8th, 2015).

Jun, J. & Worth, H. (2010). An Overview of China's HIV Epidemic. In J.Jun & H. Worth (Eds.) HIV in China: Understanding the Social Aspects of the Epidemic. Sydney: UNSW Press, pp. 13-41.

Kawachi, I. & Kennedy, B. P. (1997). Health and Social Cohesion: Why Care about Income Inequality? British Medical Journal, 314, pp. 1037-1040.

Kennedy, B., Kawachi, I., & Prothrow-Stith, D. (1996). Income Distribution and Mortality: Test of the Robin Hood Index in the United States. British Medical Journal, 312, pp. 1004-1007.

Lee, K. & Zwi, A. (2003). A Global Political Economy Approach to AIDS: Ideology, Interests and Implications. In K. Lee (Ed.) Health Impacts of Globalization. Towards Global Governance. Hampshire-New York: Palgrave Macmillan.

Lee, K. (2003). Globalization and Health. An Introduction. New York: Palgrave Macmillan.

Lee, K. (2004). Globalisation: What is it and how does it affect health? The Medical Journal of Australia, 180 (4), pp. 156-158. (https://www.mja.com.au/journal/2004/180/4/globalisation-what-it-and-how-does-it-affect-health, accessed on July 19th, 2015).

Lee, K. (2005). Global Social Change and Health. In K. Lee & J. Collin (Eds.) Global Change and Health. New York: Open University Press/ McGraw-Hill Education, pp. 13-27.

Lie, R. (2003). Spaces of Intercultural Communication: An Interdisciplinary Introduction to Communication, Culture, and Globalizing/Localizing Identities. New Jersey: Hampton Press, Inc.

MacBride, S. (1980). Many voices, one world. Communication and society. Today and tomorrow (S. MacBride Ed.) Paris: UNESCO.

MacLachan, M. (1997). Culture and Health. Chichester-New York-Weinheim-Brisbane-Singapore-Toronto: John Wiley & Sons.

Malikhao, P. (2007). HIV/AIDS Prevention Strategies in Two Thai Communities: Buddhist and Christian. Ph.D. Thesis, Brisbane: University of Queensland, Australia.

Malikhao, P. (2012). Sex in the Village. Culture, Religion and HIV/AIDS in Thailand. Southbound & Silkworm Publishers: Penang-Chiang Mai, 238pp. (ISBN: 978-983-9054-55-2).

Malikhao, P. (2013 a). Communication for Development and Sustainability. Media Development, 3, pp. 1-5.

Malikhao, P. (2013 b). Understanding the Spread of HIV/AIDS in Thailand. In J. Servaes (Ed.) Sustainability, Participation and Culture in Communication. Intellect/University of Chicago Press: Bristol/Chicago, pp.273-292.

Marmot, M. & Bell, R. (2006). The Socioeconomically Disadvantage. In B. S. Levy & V. W. Side (Ed.) Social Injustice and Public Health. Oxford-New York: Oxford University Press.

Martin, J. N. & Nakayama, T. K. (2004). Intercultural Communication in Contexts. McGraw Hill: Boston.

Moore, M., Gould, P. & Keary, B. (2003). Global Urbanization and Impact on Health. International Journal of Hygiene and Environmental Health, 206, pp. 269-278.

Nash, K. (2000). Contemporary Political Sociology. London: Blackwell Publishers.

Nestle, M. (2006). What to Eat. New York: North Point Press.

Nestle, M. (2013). Food Politics. How the Food Industry Influences Nutrition and Health. Berkeley-Los Angeles-London: University of California Press.

Nestle, M. (2007). Food Politics. How the Food Industry Influences Nutrition and Health. Berkeley-Los Angeles-London: University of California Press.

Nisbett, R. E. (2003). The Geography of Thought: How Asians and Westerners Think Differently and Why. New York-London-Toronto-Sydney-Singapore: The Free Press.

Perrings, C. (2014). Our Uncommon Heritage. Biodiversity Change, Ecosysem Services, and Human Well-being. Cambridge: Cambridge University Press.

Pollard, T. M. (2008). Western Diseases. An Evolutionary Perspective. Cambridge: Cambridge University Press.

Powell, J. L. & Steel, R. (2011). Revisiting Appadurai: Globalizing Scapes in a Globalized World-The Pervasiveness of Economic and Cultural Power. International Journal of Innovative Interdisciplinary Research 1, December 1: 74-80.

Ruiz-Nunez, B., Pruimboom, L., Dijck-Brouwer, D.A. J., Muskiet, F. A. J. (2013). Lifestyle and Nutritional Imbalances Associated with Western Diseases: Causes and Consequences of Chronic Systemic Low Grade Inflammation in an Evolutionary Context. The Journal of Nutritional Biochemistry 24(7), pp. 1183-1201. (doi: 10.1016/j/jnutbio.2013.02.009).

Schneider, M. (2006). Introduction to Public Health. Boston: Jones and Bartlett Publishers.

Scholte, J. A. (2005). Globalization: A Critical Introduction. Basingstoke: Palgrave Macmillan.

Summerfield, L. M. (2012). Nutrition, Exercise, & Behavior. An Integrated Approach to Weight Management. Belmont, CA: Wadsworth.

The Levin Institute-The State University of New York (2014). Globalization 101. (http://www.globalization101.org/diseases-go-global/, accessed on Jan 11th, 2015).

Thompson, J. (1995). The Media and Modernity. A Social Theory of the Media. Cambridge: Polity Press.

Wermuth, L. (2003). Global Incquality and Human Needs. Boston: Pearson Education, Inc.

Wickrama, K. A. S., Lorenz, F. O., Conger, R. D. & Elder, G. H. (1997). Linking Occupational Conditions to Physical Health through Material, Social and Interpersonal Processes. Journal of Health and Social Behavior. 38 (4): 363-375.

Wilkinson, R. & Pickett, K. (2009). The Spirit Level: Why Equality is Better for Everyone. London: Allen Lane.

Wilkinson, R. G. (1997). Health Inequalities: Relative or Absolute Material Standards? British Medical Journal, 314(7080), pp. 591-595.

Williams, D. R. (1990). Socioeconomic Differntials in Health: A Review and Redirection. Social Psychology Quarterly 53 (2): 81-99.

Yach, D. & Beaglehole, R. (2004). Globalization of Risks for Chronic Diseases Demands Global Solutions. In R. L. Harris & M. Seid (Eds.) Globalization and Health. Leiden & Boston: Brill, pp. 213-233.

Yach, D. (2006). Chronic Disease. In B. S. Levy & V. W. Sidel (eds.) Social Injustice and Public Health. Oxford-New York: Oxford University Press, pp. 253-276.

Websites

Centers for Disease Control and Prevention (CDC)

CDC 2010

http://www.cdc.gov/h1n1flu/cdcresponse.htm, accessed on September 3rd, 2015.

CDC 2014 a

http://www.cdc.gov/flu/avianflu/h7n9-virus.htm, accessed on July

CDC 2015

http://www.cdc.gov/coronavirus/mers/index.html, accessed on September 4th, 2015.

EndocrineWeb 2015

http://www.endocrineweb.com/conditions/type-1-diabetes/what-insulin, accessed on September 5th, 2015.

International Agency for Research on Cancer (IARC, WHO, 2013)

http://www.iarc.fr/en/media-centre/iarcnews/pdf/pr221_E.pdf, accessed on September 12th, 2015.

MedicineNet.com 2015

http://www.medicinenet.com/aerobic_exercise/article.htm, accessed on September 5th, 2015.

NASA 2015

http://climate.nasa.gov/effects/, accessed on September 15, 2015.

National Geographic 2015

http://environment.nationalgeographic.com/environment/global-warming/ozone-depletion-overview/depletion-overview/, accessed on September 15th, 2015.

News.softpedia.com 2007

http://news.softpedia.com/news/Top-10-Infectious-Diseases-That-Have-Killed-Most-People-70741.shtml, accessed on January 29th, 2016.

PsychCentral 2015

http://psychcentral.com/lib/obesity-and-mental-health/, accessed on September 11th, 2015.

Public Broadcasting Station (PBS) 2014

http://www.pbs.org/newshour/updates/diseases-thought-eradicated-reappear-u-s/, accessed on September 4th, 2015.
The College of Physicians of Philadelphia 2015
http://www.historyofvaccines.org/content/articles/disease-eradication, accessed on July 22nd, 2015.
The Medical Journal of Australia
https://www.mja.com.au/journal/2004/180/4/globalisation-what-it-and-how-does-it-affect-health, accessed on July 19th, 2015.
U.S. Environmental Protection Agency (EPA)
1). EPA 1991
http://www.epa.gov/iaq/pdfs/sick_building_factsheet.pdf, accessed on September 12th, 2015.
2). EPA2013
http://www.epa.gov/wastes/hazard/tsd/pcbs/pubs/about.htm, accessed on September 9th, 2015.
3). EPA 2015
http://www.epa.gov/climatechange/ghgemissions/gases.html, accessed on September 15th, 2015.
WebMD
1). WebMD 2013
http://www.webmd.com/brain/mad-cow-disease-basics?page=3#1, accessed on September 4th, 2015.
2). WebMD2015 a
http://www.webmd.com/sleep-disorders/features/important-sleep-habits?page=2, accessed on September 11th, 2015.
World Health Organization (WHO)
WHO 2015 a (non communicable disease)
http://www.who.int/mediacentre/factsheets/fs355/en/, accessed Jan 11th, 2015
WHO 2015 b antimicrobial drug resistance
http://www.who.int/csr/disease/OP_AMR_FINAL.pdf?ua=1, accessed on July 22nd, 2015.
WHO 2015 c top ten cause of death
http://who.int/mediacentre/factsheets/fs310/en/index1.html, accessed on September 4th, 2015.

Chapter 4

HEALTH DETERMINANTS FROM ANTHROPOLOGICAL AND SOCIOLOGICAL PERSPECTIVES

ABSTRACT

This chapter focuses on health inequalities, which can be innate and constructed by the socials. Basic demographic attributes that contribute to health inequalities are explained. Health inequalities caused by socioeconomic, cultural and environmental determinants will be reviewed. The knowledge of medical anthropology and sociology can be used to understand the context of health. Health communicators could use this knowledge to devise their strategies to communicate on/about health effectively.

Keywords: health inequalities, gender, culture, beliefs, religious culture, world view, epigenetics, health care services

INTRODUCTION

As discussed in the previous chapters, health is a dynamic interaction among many determinants. To understand the context of health, it is important that health communication scholars have a basic understanding of two distinctive social science fields: Sociology and Anthropology. In *Chapter 2* of this book, the reader learned that some communication theories are based on social psychology, some on sociology, or other disciplines. This chapter explains how sociology and anthropology can assist health communication practitioners to plan, execute and sustain community health.

Sociology helps the study of health communication to understand the social construction of health. As discussed in the previous chapters, health is not only related to the biomedical aspect, the extrinsic health determinants are complex and have impact on our well-being. They are healthcare policies, political economy, social status, social class, health education, social support, bioethics, environment, and so forth. Medical sociology is a more specific area of sociology that is used to understand that some sorts of illness are caused by social patterns and social interactions. It is an application of the study of social science research on health and healthcare. It includes the study of medicine as a profession; the role of sickness and illness experiences; social construction of illness and medical knowledge, inclusive medicalization; sociological epidemiology; and sociological study of healthcare services as organizations (Bird, Conrad & Fremont 2000: 2). This area of study is different from medical anthropology which studies health, illness, and healing across the board of human societies and over the life course with an emphasis on how members of the community behave, express and articulate, access, and manage their resources within the community power structure (Janzen 2002: 2). Medical anthropology looks at cultures, both material aspects (such as artefacts and lifestyles), and immaterial aspects (such as the meaning of signs of illness and suffering), to unfold and interpret health seeking and health restoring (Janzen 2002: 2). A critical medical anthropology is "a perspective which views health issues within the context of encompassing political and economic forces that pattern human relationships, shape social behaviors, condition collective experiences, re-order local ecologies, and situate cultural meanings, including forces of institutional, national, and global scale" (Baer, Singer & Susser 1997: 3-4).

Both sociological and anthropological research is very useful to assess the socioeconomic, cultural, and political context of individual and community health, healthcare services, and medical traditions. Communicating on health for sustainable development should start from the realization that health inequalities are caused by individual attributes, social ascription, and general socioeconomic, cultural and environmental conditions. Knowing both the context and the content of health helps health communication practitioners to assess the sustainability of healthcare services and health campaigns.

HEALTH INEQUALITIES

Health inequality means that not everyone has an equal chance to enjoy the minimum standard of healthy living, based on access to good quality early childhood development, education and employment; empowerment to take control over one's life; a political voice; and the ability to participate in decision-making processes (WHO Europe 2015: 63-64). The socioeconomic position of an individual, family, communities, regions, and societies is a reason that health inequalities exist and persist (Robert & House 2000: 80). As reported in *Chapter 3*, living in a poor socioeconomic position prevent people from accessing nutritious foods, decent housing and sanitation, proper schooling, regular health and dental check-ups, preventive care, healthcare, a safe neighborhood, meaningful job, leisure time and sports. Lacking quality of life increases stress and that may lead to tobacco addiction, and alcohol, drug and substance abuse, domestic violence, and poor mental health. In *Chapter 3*, I refer to "affluenza," which is defined as a painful, contagious, socially transmitted condition of overload, debt, anxiety, and waste resulting from the dogged pursuit of more of those who occupy a high socioeconomic position (de Graaf, Wann, & Naylor 2014). To elaborate on this mental disorder, it is a state of confusion that one fails to distinguish between wants and needs (Hamilton and Denniss 2005: 7, 14-15). People are emotionally insecure; feel anxious, bored, isolated, and alienated. They want to consume more and experiment more. The key characteristics for people with affluenza is thinking that nothing bad can happen to them and that can lead to addiction to alcohol, mood-altering drugs, and sex (Northbound treatment services 2013).

The socio-demographic (e.g., age, ethnicity, gender, and location) together with the socioeconomic status (SES), the social environmental and medical (i.e., residential characteristics, occupational environment, social support, social/professional hierarchy, and access to health care), the psychological and behavioral (i.e., psychological distress, personality factors, health promoting behaviors, and health damaging behaviors), and physiological (cardiovascular, immune, muscular, endocrine, height, and weight) determine health and illness of a person (Anderson & Armstead 1995: 213-225).

Not only is the socioeconomic position of individuals and families associated with health at an individual level, the socioeconomic characteristics of communities, regions, and societies can also play mediating roles to the individual level of health. Sociological research done in this field recognizes the interplay of basic demographic attributes: race, gender, and age with the social stratification on health outcomes. These attributes will be addressed next.

Basic Demographic Attributes and Health Inequalities

Health gaps within demographic variables such as gender, age, and race or ethnicity are wide due to innate differences between genders, age groups, or genes in each race. The differences are modulated by other socioeconomic and environmental determinants. Let's focus on the basic attributes first, to see what differences they make about health.

Gender-Based Inequalities in Health

Women live with diseases but men die from them. That statement can be derived from much research that has been undertaken on the life course of different genders for many decades. Health inequality between genders is partly innate. Factual data show women outlive men in all parts of the world by five to six years, disregarding of whether both genders live in developed or developing countries (WHO 2014). The factors that help explain why women have longer life expectancy are fivefold: first, biological factors—differences between hormones and DNA of male and female sex; second, evolutionary factors—biological adaptation of the females over a long period of time to reproduce offspring; third, societal factors—the interplay between physical health and the social conditions; forth, psychological factors—this is to explain the addiction to tobacco, alcohol and substance abuse among males and females; and fifth, from the dynamic interaction of the three aforementioned factors.

From biological explanations, Perls and Fretts (1988: 100-103) report that in part sex hormones – testosterone in males and estrogen in females --, play a role in the longevity of females over males. They explain further that during the onset of puberty, males are likely to die three times more than females. The testosterone hormone that men excrete after puberty increases the low-density lipoprotein (known as bad cholesterol) and decreases the level of high-density lipoprotein (known as good cholesterol). This puts men at greater risk of cardiovascular diseases than women. On the contrary, estrogen that females excrete increases good cholesterol and decreases bad cholesterol. It is an antioxidant that helps delay aging, neural and vascular damage, and onset of Alzheimer's disease. Thus, physically men are more inclined to die of heart disease and stroke than women.

Moreover, Perls and Fretts (1988: 100-103) state that menstruation in females may contribute to their longevity as premenopausal women have 20 percent less blood in their body than men, and a lower iron load that could form oxygen radicals. The lower iron load leads to slower aging. Also women have a lower metabolic rate than men and that makes it less vulnerable for their cells to break down.

Giddens, Duneier, Appelbaum, and Carr (2014: 473) report genetics factors that help explain why the number of male fetus miscarriages, male infant deaths, and male death at all ages is above that of women because of congenital abnormalities and the poorer cardiopulmonary systems of males. The culprit lies in the sex chromosomes. Males have XY sex chromosomes while females have XX ones. The X chromosome carries more genetic information and defects that can lead to physical anomalies than the Y. The female thus has an extra X chromosome to override the possible abnormal one, while the male who has a defective X chromosome, will manifest the symptoms as they have no extra X chromosome as female do.

From an evolutionary explanation, the longevity of women is part of natural selection for fecundity, so that the women could rear the offspring and protect them from early childhood mortality rates (Perls & Fretts 1988: 100-103).

From sociological explanations, stressors from living and working in society affect the mental health of both men and women. The social construction of gender seems to affect the mental health of females more than males. Married males were reported to have better mental health than single males but married females seem to have worse mental health (Rieker and Bird 2000: 103). Rieker and Bird (2000: 102-103) report that females tend to have a higher rate of depression than males because of lower rewarding jobs and overloading housework and work outside of the house. Being caregivers of children as a gender role reduces the female's ability to take care of themselves properly. That is the cause of mild physical illnesses among females. Males, as expected in their gender role to be breadwinners, were found to have higher rates of substance abuse, smoking and alcohol from stress, than females. That makes that males die earlier than females from cancer and cardiovascular diseases. During the past three decades more females have taken on the masculine role of working and health risk-taking behaviors, such as drinking and smoking; they have become more likely to suffer from men's diseases as well. There were no gender differences in death rate from smoking, reported Perls and Fretts (1988: 103).

From psychological explanations, this is used to address stress coping behavior between genders. Men are found more likely to use problem-focused strategies while women use emotion-focused strategies in dealing with stressors, regardless of occupation or education (Sarafino 2006: 122).

From mixed explanations, there are always crossing effects between biological factors, evolutionary, sociological, and psychological ones that impinge on individual health risk-taking behaviors differently. Let's take smoking as an example. Psychosocial research found that a teen who smokes tends to have at least one parent who smokes or felt peer pressure to smoke (Sarafino 2006: 176). From world statistics, 31 percent of males compared with 6 percent of females smoked daily in 2014, compared with 41 percent of males and 10 percent of females in 1980. The gender gap of smoking has been narrowing because larger numbers of males (in stead of women) stopped smoking (BBC 2014). The changing role of females in the society that causes stress may be one explanation why females smoke more. The fact that poorer people smoke more (BBC 2014) indicates that the low socioeconomic status induces stress as well. This may be enhanced by biological factors, as it was found that nicotine addiction runs in the family. Nicotine transmitted from mother to baby during the pregnancy period may make the child more susceptible to nicotine addiction (Kandel, Wu & Davies

1994). Another biological research found that smoking can reduce stress temporarily, but may increase it in the long run (Parrott 1999). All of the factors combined would help explain gender-based smoking addiction.

Age-Based Inequalities in Health

Aging is a process that combines the following development clocks: biological clock refers to the physical body; psychological, refers to the mind including one's mental, emotional, and cognitive capabilities; and social, which refers to cultural norms, values, and role expectations related to age (Giddens, Duneier, Appelbaum & Carr 2014: 272). Different diseases occur throughout the life course of an individual. During childhood, diseases such as chicken pox, measles, mumps, rubella, whooping cough occur. During adulthood, diseases such as obesity, hypertension, diabetes type II, fatty liver; maternal mortality; occupational injuries could occur. During old age, flu and pneumonia, Alzheimer's, dementia, and cancer, for instance, could occur.

As people grow older, the agility and vigor of the physical and psychological aspect will decline. But that does not mean that the aging process cannot be delayed with a healthy lifestyle. Some diseases that occur most during the childhood can be prevented by vaccination, such as Diphtheria-Tetanus-Polio. Some diseases occurring during adulthood can be prevented by vaccination as well (such as flu, human papilloma virus, and so forth). But certain chronic diseases such as cardiovascular diseases, diabetes mellitus; and cancer can be prevented by eating less quantities but more in quality food, such as choosing to eat a largely plant-based diet, eating less red meat, less high-fat dairy products, less fried or processed foods; or eating more foods low in fat, saturated fat, cholesterol, sugar, and salt (Nestle 2013: 31-50, 77). Living a healthy lifestyle means eating right, controlling stress up to a low or modest level, and exercising regularly and vigorously. Together with advances in medical technology it could delay the onset of the biological ageing process (Giddens, Duneir, Appelbaum & Carr 2014: 273).

The stages of aging – childhood, adolescence, adulthood, and old age – are socially constructed and vary across cultures. For instance, the new paradigm of childhood has shifted from becoming skilled and knowledgeable members of society to active social participants who are able to construct and give meanings to one's own lives, cultures, and relationships (Giddens & Sutton 2012). By the same token, the elderly and old age terms are also socially constructed. Aging has different meanings across cultures. Giddens, Duneier, Appelbaum and Carr (2014: 278) state that the young old (ages 65-74), the old old (ages 75 to 84), and the oldest old (ages 85 and older) are different in degree of independence, health, activity and engagement, and economic status. The older one becomes, the less independent, the less healthy, the less active and engaged, and the poorer one becomes.

The retirement age is also different from one country to another. The retirement age in Belgium has shifted from 65 to 67 years, while the retirement age in Thailand is 60 years. In many countries it is gender-dependent, meaning that often women can retire earlier than man. When people retire they change officially from an active to inactive work status and, by doing so, earn less. Some people live on their pension funds; some on savings. The retiree financial situation depends on their occupation. Income inequality among age groups comes into the picture. Gender may mediate the effect more, as women live longer than men but, in general, earn less than men. Also ethnicity could be a mediating variable as well. For instance, older Caucasian Americans, in general, earn more than older people from ethnic minority groups

(Giddens & Sutton 2012). Less income, in general, would indicate less disease prevention, poorer nutrition, less frequent check-ups, and less quality care unless the person is a citizen of the Western-European countries where governments still provide universal healthcare.

Ethnicity and Race-Based Inequalities in Health

Pollard (2008: 55-70) reports that certain ethnic groups possess genotypes that are accountable for metabolic syndromes such as type 2 diabetes, hypertension, and obesity, and subsequently coronary heart disease, as a result of genetic adaptation to control the metabolism during the times of food abundance and scarcity along the evolutionary path. When these people changed their lifestyles to a more sedentary one and eat more fat and refined carbohydrate, like people in the Western world, they would develop insulin resistance. Insulin resistance means that the body cannot respond properly to the insulin it makes and that causes the rise of the sugar level in blood overtime (WebMD 2015 c). The people would subsequently develop an onset of metabolic syndromes. These peoples are, for instance, the Maoris in New Zealand, the Micronesians, the Native Americans in the US, and the Aborigines in Australia.

Pollard (2008: 54) also reports medical anthropological research on people who migrated from South Asia to the UK and the US and had to change their dietary patterns to higher fat and higher refined carbohydrates. These people were found tending to develop insulin resistance. Consequently, they tended to have onset type 2 diabetes and coronary heart diseases.

Research confirms that Asian people tend to have a higher prevalence of diabetes than Europeans due to the fact that they tend to have a higher proportion of body fat for the same BMI as that of Europeans (Pollard 2008: 160).

Those are gestational discrepancies in health caused by race and ethnicity. However, other determinants that mediate this can make the ethnicity-based gap of health equity even wider. For instance, Western people eat a diet low in fibers and high in protein and fat. This was found the cause for chronic non-communicable diseases among Western people, such as gastrointestinal, cardiovascular, metabolic, etc. (Campbell & Chen 1994: 67-108). Other determinants such as racism and poverty would aggravate the racial inequalities in health. It was found that African Americans have higher hypertension rates than White Americans partly due to poverty and racism (Pollard 2008: 72). The high rate of teen pregnancy among Hispanic Americans is conditioned by growing up in poverty, having parents with low education, a low performance at school, and growing up in a single-parent family (CDC 2014 b). It is found that the high HIV/AIDS prevalence in Africa is due to poverty as well (HIV/AIDS electronic library 2015).

Apart from demographic attributes, the interaction of socioeconomic, cultural and environmental determinants affects health inequalities also, as will be addressed next.

Socioeconomic, Cultural and Environmental Determinants' Impact on Health Inequalities

As explained in *Chapter 3*, globalization, visible in various external factors, is partly responsible for health inequalities. However, internal factors cannot be neglected as health inequalities are maintained and upheld by dynamic interactions of many social determinants, such as the social status, religious culture and belief systems, living and working environment, medical and pharmaceutical industry, health care services, and food industry.

Social Status

Social status used to be understood as social class. Indicators of class include wealth and property, and income. Wealth and property are what has been accumulated for generations for some people, and that is different from income. Wealth can come from stock holdings for business people, inheritance for the old rich, sponsorship for sportspersons, etc. Occupation determines income. Education also determines occupation. All of the afore-mentioned indicate class. Class structure can be divided in the US as capitalist class, upper-middle class, middle class, working class, working poor, and underclass. Gilbert and Kahl (1982) and Gilbert (2008) report the American class structure as follows:

- "Capitalist class: investors, heirs, and executives, typically with prestigious university education and annual family income over $2 million, mostly from assets.
- Upper-middle class: high-level managers, professionals, midsize business owners with college education, most often with advanced degrees with family income of $120,000 or more.
- Middle class: low-level managers, semiprofessionals, some persons in sales and skilled crafts, foremen and supervisors with at least high school education, usually some college, technical training, or apprenticeship and family incomes of about $55,000.
- Working class: high school-educated operatives, clerical workers, most retail salesclerks, routinized assembly and factory workers, and related "blue-collar" employees with family incomes of about $35,000.
- Working poor: poorly paid service workers and laborers, operatives, and clerical workers in low-wage sectors, usually with some high school and family incomes of around $22,000.
- Underclass: persons with erratic job histories and weak attachment to the formal labor force, unemployed or able to find only seasonal or part-time work, dependent on temporary or informal employment or some form of social assistance, and with typical family income of $12,000."

In other countries, the categorizations can be less sophisticated and split into an upper, middle, and lower class. Social status covers a broader range than social class; it includes education, employment, work, and economic status (Mirowsky, Ross & Reynolds 2000: 48-49). How each component affects health will be explained next.

Not only good education does benefit personal development in hygiene, and facilitates access to knowledge about diseases and prevention, it also provides access to meaningful employment, work and habitat in a nonhazardous environment. It is an indicator of good social support, good occupation, and good income which, in turn, boosts up self-esteem, sense of power, sense of self-control and emotional stability, job autonomy and job satisfaction, the absence of economic hardship, and a possibility to have a healthy lifestyle: smoke less, exercise more, drink moderately, have regular health check-ups (Mirowsky, Ross

& Reynolds 2000: 50-56). Mothers with more education are more likely to have received prenatal care than less educated mothers. Sarafino (2006: 158) reports individuals from lower social status are more likely to "be born with very low birth weight; die in infancy or in childhood; have poorer overall health and develop a long-standing illness in adulthood; and experience days of restricted activity because of illness."

The "health gradient" descriptive model, which linearizes the socioeconomic status (or SES) and health outcomes, can be used to (partially) explain that high level of income, education, and occupation have some association with lower death rates (Anderson & Armstead 1995: 213-215). To elaborate, low income people and paupers face a short life expectancy at birth as they have less access to appropriate healthcare, nutrition, living conditions including sanitary, and later in life they are more prone to chronic stress because of unstable job or unemployment prospects.

Race and ethnic inequality in the world and in some countries such as the US, Australia, South Africa, Malaysia, etc. have an impact on the inequality in the social status of the majority and the ethnic minorities, be it Native Americans, or aborigines, or African Americans, Africans or Chinese, and so forth. The control of the majority over the minorities in each nation can be called internal colonialism (Blauner 1972). That results in labor exploitation, inferiority, and lower social standing of the minorities. Race as well as gender is socially constructed. Gender inequality can be seen in almost every society. An easy indicator is the lower earning of females than that of males for the same white-collar job. All of these factors make the social standing of a person complicated. Health inequality among different social classes ensues. Inequality of health can be observed among nations as well. Sernau (2014: 61-62) reports that in most developed countries life expectancy at birth is about 80 percent while in the poorest countries about 50 percent; life expectancy reflects life style, diet, and health behaviors that make people live longer.

Religious Culture, Belief Systems, and Cultures

Culture is related to both material and non-material aspects. The material aspect concerns artefacts, heroes, and tangible products such as CDs, DVDs, films, etc. The non-material aspect is the socially constructed and subjective characteristics of a culture. Brown (1995: 8-9) explains different elements of culture at three levels, starting from the shallow, the middle, and the deepest level, which interact among one another. Manifestations of culture are artefacts; language; behaviour patterns in the form of rites, rituals, ceremonies and celebrations; norms of behaviour; heroes; symbols and symbolic action; beliefs, values and attitudes; ethical codes; basic assumptions; and history. The shallowest level of culture is artefacts: stories, myths, jokes, metaphors, rites, rituals and ceremonies; heroes and symbols. The middle level of culture is beliefs, values and attitudes. The deepest one is basic assumptions that concern the environment, reality, human nature, human activity and human relationship.

Another framework of culture, useful for analysing culture, cultural diversities, cultural differences and similarities, is the one that Servaes (1999: 12) has developed. He outlines four interrelated analytical components: a worldview (*Weltanschauung*), a value system, a system of symbolic representations, and a social-cultural organizational system. These four elements of culture are interrelated (Servaes 1999: 12). The first two elements are the immaterial parts of culture that can be manifested through the last two elements.

Servaes' (1999) definition – culture is a dynamic factor that can condition change in society and a way to assess the change in worldview and cultural values is through the investigation of the symbolic interactions and representations, and the social organization system — fits in the multiplicity paradigm he proposed in 1989. In a nutshell, the multiplicity paradigm calls for an interpretive or critical approach of social science, together with an interdisciplinary approach, to study the holistic influences of development, culture, social change and participatory communication. In considering globalization and the emergence of global messages at a local level, scholars emphasize an interdisciplinary approach (Geertz 1983, Giddens 1990, Lie 2003: 109), in which culture plays an important part (Robertson 1992), and in which the global is linked to the local (Sztompka 1993). The interpretive approach of the Social Science framework for intercultural communication studies can be summarized from Yashitake's (2004: 34) description as the understanding of the lifeworld through dialogue that requires intersubjective relations between the observed and the observer. For the critical approach of this social science framework, Yashitake (2004: 34) sees it as "a defense against the invasion of system into the lifeworld and/or as empowerment of the oppressed." The critical approach seems to be an antidote for the interpretive approach in which any intrusion in the systemization and rationalization of a particular culture is being investigated and interpreted. It implies the realization of power embedded in the interrelations among race, gender, class and sexuality in the construction of culture.

MacLachlan (1997: 93-94) reports that the cultural background of a person influences the experience of suffering at many levels: form, expression, and a consequence of suffering. To elaborate, a Chinese may suffer stress in the form of ache and pain while a German may suffer stress in the form of pessimism and a poor self-concept. Expressions of stress can be private (keep it to oneself), or public (share with other people), depending on culture. Consequences of suffering may differ in different cultures such as help, sympathy, frustration, anger, etc., each of which influenced by the socials. Culture-bound syndromes exist in both the Eastern and Western world. Hughes (1985) in MacLachlan (1997: 86) indicates that some cultures have a unique sickness. For example: "Bebanian, found in Bali, where a person may suddenly break into tears and attempts to run away from their present situation. They will try to fight off anybody who tries to stop them. Ultimately they collapse with exhaustion and subsequently have no memory for these events." MacLachlan (1997: 87) further reports Western culture-bound syndromes which include anorexia nervosa, type A behavior[13], Obesity, agoraphobia[14], shoplifting, and exhibitionism or flashing.

Different cultures affect an individual's psychology, pain expression, discussion of emotional problems, and definition and diagnosis of mental illness. This also includes the healing practices and the support system from family. Galanti (2008) discusses the differences in different cultures in healthcare extensively. Basic anthropological concepts such as worldview, values, emic[15] and etic[16] , and discusses topics such as pain, birth, end of

---

[13] Type A behavior is most commonly exhibited by adult males who try to multi-task against time pressure to meet deadlines. They behave aggressively, impatiently, and competitively (MacLachlan 1997: 87).

[14] Agoraphobia is a fear of leaving a restricted area. The person exhibits mood disturbance and panicking (MacLachlan 1997: 86).

[15] The emic approach is the insider approach meaning that studying culture from a perspective of the insider of a community (study.com 2015).

[16] The etic approach is studying culture with existing theories and perspective originated from outside of the culture (study.com 2015).

life, mental health and so forth to illustrate that actually health, life course events, and illnesses are partly socially constructed.

Worldview is also a part of the construction of culture. It is directly influenced by beliefs and religion. Berger and Luckmann discuss in 'The Social Construction of Reality' (1966) the interaction between thinking and action. Socialization within a tradition and culture shapes an individual's thinking, and at the same time, this internalized form is reflected in the manifestation of culture (Holm 1997: 75). This model stresses the importance of religion, as it provides a symbolic universe which explains birth, life, and death, as well as providing the individual with an identity. Religion explains the world through myths and legends and also through rational discourses. Therefore, Robertson (1972: 47) defines *religious culture* as "... a set of beliefs and symbols (and values deriving there from) pertaining to a distinction between an empirical and a super-empirical, transcendent reality; the affair of the empirical being subordinated in significance to the non-empirical."

Religion provides spiritual well-being. It affects the way people give meaning and respond to the signs and symptoms of illness, treatment, and the healing process (Spector 2000: 123). The birth and death rituals of each religion practiced in each country are different and some rituals cause health inequalities. For instance, in Chad, where 44 percent of the population is Muslims, female circumcision will be performed at birth.

Spector (2000: 144-150) reports that certain religious beliefs can affect therapy. For instance, Roman Catholics, Jehovah's Witnesses, Bah'I followers, and Christian Science followers prohibit abortion, while Muslims accept it. Some religious beliefs prohibit euthanasia (e.g., Baha'I, Christian Science, Mennonite, and Seventh-Day Adventists). The Jehovah's Witnesses are forbidden to receive blood and blood products, and are not allowed to donate organs.

Duhigg (2013: 68-71) reports how Alcoholics Anonymous (AA) has helped change about 2.1 million alcoholic people to achieve sobriety each year. Bill Wilson, the founder of AA and an agnostic, experienced that some alcoholics put their lives in the hand of God and could get out of the addictive loop. Thus, the AA steps of treatment to sobriety include spirituality. Apart from spirituality, the effect of the peer group as a support group also helps alcoholics change their old habits.

In a multi-cultural context, knowledge of many cultures, religious beliefs, and health behaviors of people in different cultures helps to empathize with people whom we are communicating with. It is known that religious beliefs have a lot of impact on people's worldviews or how people see the world.

A good communicator should not be ethnocentric—thinking that one's own culture and practices are the standard to judge other people's culture as inferior. Therefore, another definition of culture, which is useful for health communication, is the one presented by Agyeman's (2013):

> "(Culture is) predicated on differences and on otherness, and is a complex, dynamic, and embodied set of realities in which people (re)create identities, meanings, and values. Overlaying this is the reality of hybrid or multiple cultural and group affiliations. In this sense, no one person can be reduced to one single or fixed cultural form of identity."

Cultural relativism is an assumption that there is no superiority among cultures and we should not compare cultures in terms of values or merits (Hall 1959). This assumption is not universally accepted as many communities still stick to the idea that their way of life is better than others, which is called ethnocentrism (Mohammed 2011: 5). It is the tendency to judge "the other" in terms of our own experiences and expectations (Mohammed 2011: 5). Stereotyping is a way that one makes up a mental picture of groups, and their supposed characteristics, and one evaluates individuals from each group according to that mental picture, which can be a distorted view (Gannon 2008: 36).

Everyone deserves respect and humanity. One way to get rid of one's ethnocentricity is to travel abroad and spend some time in a different culture to see that peoples have different lifestyles, opinions, and ways to healing body and soul. Cultural relativism in health communication is a way to scrub off one's own ethnocentricity, prejudice and stereotyping for a better, healthier world.

Living and Working Environment

Living and working environment are related to socioeconomic status. Living in a decaying neighborhood induces depression. If a neighborhood is not safe to walk around in, it is difficult for the people to enjoy outdoor life. Moreover, if there are no sports facilities or a park for recreation, it is hard to have a healthy and fit lifestyle for the have-nots. Crowded housing and non-hygienic sanitation can cause respiratory diseases such as Severe Acute Respiratory Syndrome or SARS.

The case of SARS in Hong Kong is a lesson to learn how important the living environment is. SARS reached Hong Kong in March 2003 (Hung 2003). It spread very fast and wide. The Hong Kong public health specialists uncovered the faults in the infrastructure that helped spread the disease: the bad sanitary drainage systems of apartment buildings that allowed the mists of contaminated water to spread further (Hung 2003).

A working environment is related to education and socioeconomic status of parents. If parents are of low social class, it is hard to provide the children with a good education. Certain working environments such as working with machinery in a factory may cause injuries, or handling chemicals may cause health hazards. In developing countries, where safety regulations are lax, there is more chance that people who work in factories are exposed to toxic fumes or chemicals. When farmers in developing countries use pesticides or spray insecticides and do not wear proper masks, they inhale toxins each day. Pollution is one of the environmental problems that people in urban areas face on an almost permanent basis. Air pollution from industrial sites causes respiratory problems and cancer. Injuries from road traffics cause premature deaths. Polluted waterways from releasing sewage from industries affect people in many communities around the world. Also radioactive clouds or leaking radioactive substance and heavy metals in the sea, dumping untreated water from factories or oil spills will affect the livelihoods of people.

Medical and Pharmaceutical Industry

New maintenance therapies for chronic diseases such as diabetes, AIDS, and renal disease have prolonged the quality of life for millions of people. Advanced surgery techniques to treat previously untreatable conditions such as coronary artery bypass graft have saved many people's lives. The development of vaccines, such as the Human Papillomavirus (HPV) vaccine, has saved many people from cervical cancer. New vaccines such as Dengue vaccine and cancer vaccine are still under development. New medicines, more efficient with fewer side effects, are being introduced steadily. These can help save many lives. However, it depends on the location of the people, whether they are in the developed or developing world, to get access to these new medicines and vaccines. In general the advance of the medical and pharmaceutical industry has helped eradicate small pox. The diseases that are on the verge of being eradicated are yellow fever, Guinea worm disease, lymphatic filariasis (Elephantiasis), polio, measles, mumps, rubella, and pork tapeworm (The College of Physicians of Philadelphia 2015).

Epigenetics

Researchers found that early-life environmental and/or nutritional exposures can affect individuals' susceptibility to chronic disease development when they grow up; the impact goes deep into the DNA of a cell but not enough to change the underlying DNA sequence (Marchlewicz, Anderson & Dolinoy 2015: 4). Epigenetics is the study of changes in organisms caused by the change in phenotype[17] while those changes do not affect the genotype[18]. The diseases known as a result of aberrant epigenetics are, for instance, Alzheimer disease, schizophrenia, asthma, and autism (Marchlewicz, Anderson & Dolinoy 2015: 4). Environmental exposures can be classified into four categories: physical, chemical, nutritional, and biological. Physical exposures include radiation, noise, abuse, stress, and temperature; chemical exposures are, for instance, endocrine disrupting compounds such as bisphenol A, pesticides, persistent organic pollutants, and metals; nutritional factors such as nutrients from plants, fats, and proteins, as well as total caloric intake; and biological exposures are exposures to viruses, bacteria, and parasites, and the toxins produced and released by them.

Healthcare Services

Healthcare systems in the world differ and that causes inequalities in health among countries. According to the Public Broadcaster (PBS 2015 a) in the US, there are four basic health care systems in the world: (1) the Beveridge Model; (2) the Bismarck Model; (3) the National Health Insurance Model; and (4) the Out-of-pocket Model. Only about 40 developed countries in the world have established healthcare systems. These models are explained during the PBS documentary series Frontline, which compares the US healthcare system to five different health care systems in the world: Germany, Great Britain, Taiwan, Switzerland, and Japan (PBS 2015 b).

In the Beveridge Model, the government provides and funds the system by using tax payments. Countries that use this model are Great Britain, Hong Kong, Spain, most of Scandinavia and New Zealand. In the Bismarck Model, healthcare is provided privately by insurance funds paid by employers and employees through payroll deduction. It may look like the US system but it is fundamentally different because this system is not-for-profit and plans to cover everybody. This model is used in Germany, Japan, Belgium, the Netherlands, France, Switzerland, and to a degree in Latin America. The National Health Insurance Model uses private-sector providers funded by a government-run insurance program. This model

[17] Phenotype is defined as "the physical and psychological characteristics of an organism from both genetics and environment, or a group of organisms having like traits" (Yourdictionary.com 2015).

[18] "The definition of genotype is the genetic constitution or genetic makeup of a particular organism or group of organisms" (yourdictionary.com 2015 b).

seems to be simpler for administration and cheaper. The insurance provider can negotiate for a lower price of pharmaceutical products. Taiwan and South Korea use this model. The Out-of-pocket Model is equivalent to non-medical care for the poor and medical care for the rich, which the producers of the documentary associated the US with. The US has many different systems for many classes of people; statistics in 2014 reveals that 33 million Americans have no health insurance coverage at all (Smith & Medalia 2015:10).

Healthcare service depends on the location, whether the community is in a developed country or not. In addition, the socioeconomic status of a community does indicate whether that community has adequate services for the people in the community. That also implies the public health policy of a country.

Food Industry

The food industry is related to the marketing industry; public relations and the media; agriculture industry; politico-economy; environment; the legal system; public policy in food; nutrition and health (Nestle 2013).

As reported in the books, "Food Politics" and "What to eat" by Nestle (2007, 2006), food safety concerns contaminated food which causes illness. Examples are the use of pesticides on vegetables, antibiotics found in farm-raised fish, lead and heavy metals found in certain sea fish, radioactive substance found in seafood, mad cow disease or Bovine Spongiform Encepholopathy (BSE), hormones and antibiotics found in beef, pork, and chicken; dye pellets fed to salmons to make their flesh pink, etc. Preservatives and non-food additives in ready to eat food are abundant and that causes health hazards in the long run. Obesity in children and adults is the result of too much salt, fat, and sugar in ready-made foods and fast food. It is also questionable whether genetically modified foods, such as corn, soybeans, tomatoes, papayas, etc, – that the European Union bans but the US and other countries, especially developing countries, allow – will bring harm to human health in the long run.

CONCLUSION

In order to change one's behavior, a person needs to feel safe, feel accepted and supported by the environment. Human rights, the rights of the child, and the abolishment of all forms of discrimination must be ensured and endorsed by society. Next, education for all must be guaranteed, at least, as in the Millennial Development Goals (MDGs), for universal primary education. ('Education for all' should be replaced by 'quality education for all' to allow the inclusion of creativity, imagination, and life skill training more than rote learning or memorization).

Proper health policies and laws are a good first step. However, health professionals do need to act as social mobilizers. Participatory communication or advocacy participatory-based communication can be used to influence policy changes. Service provision should be available to support desirable behavior, such as health and educational provision, safe water supply, sanitation facilities and waste disposal, and agricultural extension services. In addition to the education system, cultural factors such as gender, widening access to political power, and socio-economic factors such as poverty and the global economy, are equally important (Spector 2000).

Health communication should not be equated with coercion. It needs the collaboration of groups of people who may differ in religion, ethnicity, lifestyles, language, etc. To overcome obstacles, a social mobilizer in health related issues should have good communication skills and be knowledgeable.

Communication as the woven thread of globalization, and tools to achieve participation for a healthy society and individuals, including health literacy, wellness/well-being, and prevention, will be discussed in relation to cultural and environmental contexts in the next chapter.

REFERENCES

Agyeman, J. (2013). *Introducing Just Sustainabilities. Policy, Planning, and Practice.* London-New York: Zed Books.

Anderson, N. B. & Armstead, C. A. (1995). Toward Understanding the Association of Socioeconomic Status and Health: A New Challenge for the Biophychosocial approach. *Psychosomatic Medicine* 57(1995): 213-225.

Baer, H. A., Singer, M. & Susser, I. (1997). *Medical Anthropology and the World System: A Critical Perspective.* Westport CT: Bergin & Garvey.

Berger, P. L. & Luckmann, T. (1966). *The Social Construction of Reality: A Treatise in the Sociology of Knowledge.* New York: Doubleday & Co.

Bird, C. E., Conrad, P., & Fremont, A. M. (2000). Medical Sociology at the Millennium. In (C. E. Bird, P. Conrad, & A. M. Fremont eds.) *Handbook of Medical Sociology* (5th Ed.) Upper Saddle NJ: Prentice-Hall, Inc., pp. 1-10.

Blauner, R. (1972). *Racial Oppression in America.* New York: Harper.

Brown, A. (1995). *Organisational Culture.* London: Pitman Publishing.

Campbell, T. C. & Chen, J. (1994). Diet and Chronic Degenerative Diseases. A Summary of Results from an Ecology Study in Rural China. In (N. J. Temple & D. P. Burkitt eds.) *Western Diseases. Their Dietary Prevention and Reversibility.* Totowa, NJ: Humana Press, pp. 67-118.

De Graaf, J., Wann, D. & Naylor, T. H. (2014). *Affluenza: how overconsumption is killing us—and how we can fight back (3rd ed.).* San Francisco: Berrett-Koehler Publishers, Inc.

Duhigg, C. (2013). *The Power of Habit. Why We Do What We Do and How to Change.* London: Random House Books.

Galanti, G. (2008). Caring for Patients from Different Cultures (4th ed.). Philadelphia: University of Pennsylvania Press.

Gannon, M. J. (2008). *Paradoxes of Culture and Globalization.* Los Angeles-London-New Delhi-Singapore: Sage Publications.

Geertz, C. (1983). *Local Knowledge.* New York: Basic Books, Inc.

Giddens, A. (1990). *The Consequence of Modernity.* Cambridge: Polity Press.

Giddens, A. & Sutton, P. W. (2012). Chapter Summary for Chapter 9 The Life Course. www.polity.co.uk/giddens7/studentresource/summaries/Student_summary_09.asp.

Giddens, A., Duneier, M., Appelbaum, R. P., & Carr, D. (2014). Introduction to Sociology. New York-London: W. W. Norton & Company, Inc.

Gilbert, D. (2008). *The American Class Structure in an Age of Growing Inequality*. (7th ed). Thousand Oaks, CA: Pine Forge.

Gilbert, D. & Kahl, J. (1982). *The American Class Structure: A New Synthesis*. Homewood, IL: Dorsey.

Hall, E. T. (1959). *The Silent Language*. New York: Doubleday.

Hamilton, C. & Denniss, R. (2005). *Affluenza. When too Much is Never Enough*. Crows Nest NSW: Allen & Unwin.

HIV/AIDS Electronic Library. (2015). http://library.unesco-iicba.org/English/HIV_AIDS/cdrom%20materials/Poverty.htm, accessed June 22, 2015.

Holm, N. (1997). An Integrated Role Theory for the Psychology of Religion: Concepts and Perspectives. In B. Spilka & D. McIntosh (Eds.), *The Psychology of Religion* (pp. 73-94). Oxford: Westview Press. http://search.ebscohost.com/login.aspx?direct=true&db=aph&AN=20921322&site=ehost-live.

Huang, Y. (2013). *Governing Health in Contemporary China*. New York: Routledge.

Hung, L. S., (2003). The SARS Epidemic in Hong Kong: What Lessons Have We Learned? *Journal of the Royal Society of Medicine*. 96(8); 2003 August, (http://www.ncbi.nlm.nih.gov/pmc/articles/PMC539564/, accessec Jan 12, 2015).

Janzen, J.M. (2002: 148). *The Social Fabric of Health*: *An Introduction to Medical Anthropology*. Boston: McGrawHill.

Kandel, D. B., Wu, P., & Davies, M. (1994). Maternal smoking during pregnancy and smoking by adolescent daughters. *American Journal of Public Health*, 84, 1407-1413.

Lie, R. (2003). *Spaces of Intercultural Communication: An Interdisciplinary Introduction to Communication, Culture, and Globalizing/Localizing Identities*. New Jersey: Hampton Press, Inc.

MacLachlan, M. (1997). *Culture and Health*. New York: John Wiley & Sons.

Marchlewicz, E. H., Anderson, O. S., & Dolinoy, D.C. (2015). Early-Life Exposures and the Epigenome. Interactions between Nutrients and the Environment. In (E. Ho & F. Domann eds.) *Nutrition and Epigenetics*. London-New York: CRC Press, pp. 3-52.

Mirowsky, J., Ross, C. & Reynolds, J. (2000). Link between Social Status and Health Status. In C. E. Bird, P. Conrad & A. M. Fremont (Eds.) *Handbook of Medical Sociology*. Upper Saddle River, N.J: Prentice-Hall, Inc., pp. 68-78.

Mohammed, S. N. (2011). *Communication and the Globalization of Culture*. Lanham-Boulder-New York-Toronto-Plymouth, UK: Lexington Books.

Nestle, M. (2013). *Food Politics. How the Food Industry Influences Nutrition and Health* (10th ed.). Berkeley-Los Angeles-London: University of California Press.

Parrott, A. C. (1999). Does cigarette smoking cause stress? *American Psychologist*, 54, 817-820.

Perls, T. T. & Fretts, R. C. (1988). Why Women Live Longer than Men. *Scientific American*, pp. 100-103.

Pollard, T. M. (2008). *Western Diseases. An Evolutionary Perspective*. Cambridge, UK: Cambridge University Press.

Rieker, P. P. & Bird, C. E. (2000). Sociological Explanations of Gender Differences in Mental and Physical Health. In In (C. E. Bird, P. Conrad, & A. M. Fremont eds.) *Handbook of Medical Sociology* (5th Ed.) Upper Saddle NJ: Prentice-Hall, Inc., pp. 98-113.

Robert, S. A. & House, J. S. (2000). Socioeconomic Inequalities in Health: An Enduring Sociological Problem. In (C. E. Bird, P. Conrad, & A. M. Fremont eds.) *Handbook of Medical Sociology* (5th Ed.) Upper Saddle NJ: Prentice-Hall, Inc., pp. 79-111.

Robertson, R. (1972). *The Sociological Interpretation of Religion*. Oxford: Basil Blackwell.

Sernau, S. (2014). *Social Inequality in a Global Age(4th ed.)*. Los Angeles-London-New Delhi-Singapore-Washington DC: Sage.

Servaes, J. (1999). *Communication for Development: One World, Multiple Cultures* (first ed.). Cresskill, New Jersey: Hampton Press, Inc.

Smith, J. C. & Medalia, C. (2015). Health Insurance Coverage in the United States: 2014. Current Population Reports. September. https://www.census.gov/content/dam/Census/library/publications/2015/demo/p60-253.pdf, accessed on February 22, 2016.

Spector, R. E. (2000). *Cultural Diversity in Health & Illness*. Upper Saddle, N.J: Prentice Hall Health.

Sztompka, P. (1993). *The Sociology of Social Change*. Cambridge, U.S.A.: Basil.

Williams, D. R. (1990). Socioeconomic Differntials in Health: A Review and Redirection. *Social Psychology Quarterly* 53 (2): 81-99.

World Health Organization Regional Office for Europe (2013). *Health 2020. A European Policy Framework and Strategy for the 21st Century*. WHO Regional Office for Europe: Denmark.

Yoshitake, M. (2004). "Research Paradigm for Dialogue among Diversities. Refinement of Methodological Pluralism." In G.-M. Chen & W. J. Starosta (eds.) Dialogue among Diversities. Washington D.C: National Communication Association.

Websites

BBC news services 2014
http://www.bbc.com/news/health-25635121, accessed on June 18th, 2015.

Centers for Disease Control and Prevention (CDC) 2014 b
http://www.cdc.gov/teenpregnancy/about/index.htm, accessed June 22, 2015.

Northbound Treatment Services 2013
http://www.livingsober.com/affluenza-drug-addiction/#.VYZyxPmqqko, accessed on June 19th, 2015.

Public Broadcasting Services (PBS)
PBS 2015 a
http://www.pbs.org/wgbh/pages/frontline/sickaroundtheworld/countries/models.html, accessed on June 24th, 2015
PBS 2015 b
http://www.pbs.org/wgbh/pages/frontline/sickaroundtheworld/, accessed June 24, 2015.

Study.com 2015
http://study.com/academy/lesson/etic-and-emic-world-views-in-anthropology.html, accessed October 14, 2015.

The College of Physicians of Philadelphia (2015).
http://www.historyofvaccines.org/content/articles/disease-eradication, accessed on June 24th, 2015.

WebMD 2015 c

http://www.webmd.com/diabetes/guide/insulin-resistance-syndrome, accessed on June 22nd, 2015.

World Health Organization (WHO) 2014
http://www.who.int/mediacentre/news/releases/2014/world-health-statistics-2014/en/, accessed on June 19th, 2015.

Yourdictionary.com 2015
2015 a
http://www.yourdictionary.com/phenotype, accessed on November 16, 2015.
2015 b
http://www.yourdictionary.com/genotype, accessed on November 16, 2015.

Chapter 5

COMMUNICATING FOR/ABOUT HEALTH FOR SUSTAINABLE DEVELOPMENT

ABSTRACT

This chapter discusses communication processes to bring about sustainability in health. Media and communication in the contemporary globalization period as related to health communication success are discussed. Rethinking about health and different approaches to health communication are explored. Communication attitude and the role of a health communicator under the framework of the multiplicity paradigm are explained. Health communication for sustainable development is defined and assessment criteria and intercultural communication competencies are presented.

Keywords: behavioral change communication, mass communication, participatory communication, Communication for structural and sustainable social change, empathy, cultural relativity, intercultural communication

INTRODUCTION

Globalization, as discussed in *Chapter 3*, is an ongoing process of passing down cross-cultural understandings via communication. Boyd-Barrett (2015: 120-121) explains seven important ways media, information, and communication industries interrelate with the globalization process. Media, information and communication industries are responsible for, first, netting global communications via the global physical infrastructure, such as wired and wireless telecommunication; second, providing a possibility of media conglomerates to operate in the neoliberal world economic order; third, being vehicles for the advertising of goods and services on the global and local scale; fourth, triggering imitation and desires for goods and services and thereby stimulating consumerism through its projection and presentation of lifestyles of others; fifth, feeding the global financial and commercial with interactive infrastructures and instruments suitable for massive electronic trading activities necessary for modern capitalism; sixth, policing and promoting ideologies and interests of neoliberalists while excluding the outliers; and seventh, supporting the surveillance society by increasing access to private eyes and intelligence. All of these show that communication technology and processes have shaped our postmodern society and affected our social interactions and values in unprecedented ways. It is fair to say there is no postmodern culture without the so-called "communication and information superhighway" and at the same time the communication process is an indispensable part of our culture. Globalization goes hand in hand with localization. Localization is the process through which the locals, in whatever boundary, pick up and adapt cultural products from the global via information and communication technologies (ICT). Through localization, the local governance, politics of leadership, administration, and jurisprudence modify or filter the influence of the global culture fostered by the global communication media on the locals and the locals interpret this foreign text and media by using their own beliefs and values (Mohammed 2011: 48-49, Lie 2003: 113). This is what Thompson (1995) calls local appropriation of culture.

Due to globalization, culture change speeded up by communications technology is evident. That means, we could observe and study how people live their life in both negative and positive ways. Negatively speaking, as discussed in *Chapter 3*, globalization brings about new kinds of diseases; biodegradation and environmental erosion such as climate change, global warming, and the extinction of some species. Positively speaking, globalization brings in new medical technology; new paths to disease prevention, alleviation, and eradication; new ways to communicate about health; and new approaches to solve environmental issues.

Fox (2012: 57-69) identifies ongoing issues and debates on health communication, such as the weak link between communication and epidemiological analysis (e.g., in polio eradication); lacking funding in the public sector; weak capacity building between the civil sector, academia, leadership, the public sector, and resources; the missing link between knowledge and behavior; the integration of IT and interdisciplinary knowledge; and most importantly, the effectiveness evaluation of any health communication program. From *Chapters 3* and *4*, we have learned that many contextual factors or determinants affect our health as well as the built-in inequalities of health in each individual. In this chapter, we will emphasize the importance of communication within a given culture. How communication cements all involving sectors and stakeholders in a participatory fashion will be explained. Also, how communication is used to advocate for funding, to enhance the collaboration among interdisciplinary experts to address health issues and to empower the stakeholders to take the health issues in their own hands will be further detailed.

Failures of health communication in the past, as described by Fox (2012: 57-69), indicate that communication as a transmission view model, emphasizing sender-message-channels-receiver-feedback, has its limitations. The 2015 World Bank report (World Bank Group 2015: 146) supports such a model by stating that informing people that there is a way to improve their health is not enough to change their health behavior; successful health communication should concern information disseminating, demonstrating and modeling health behavior, problem solving, providing social support, providing materials necessary for adoption of the health behavior, and providing a background of support through interpersonal media or the mass media. What the World Bank misses are the contextual factors that supersede, intervene, or blockade the health behavior outcomes. A holistic view of looking at the enabling environment is needed: we should see that health communication links the following components: health education; e-health and medical technology; healthcare system; market economy and advertisements that have impacts on health; pharmaceutical industry; environment; and chosen health communication strategy within a given cultural context altogether. Health education is necessary for introducing knowledge and attitudes on hygiene, wellness, well-being, health literacy, and to teach about the impact of the environment on health. Digital media technology is needed to share health information, knowledge, and practices, and strengthen participation from the audience in a two-way communication fashion. Also ICT and medical technology are important for the improvement of prevention and treatments of maladies. Communication should be used to advocate whether the government should see health as the right of all citizens to be treated in times of sickness instead of seeing health as a commodity which only benefits those who can afford to pay for health insurance. One should realize that the global market economy is being manipulated by global corporations that create predictable global consumption patterns (Mohammed 2011: 49). Next, health communicators should not neglect the impacts of advertisements from the food or pharmaceutical industry on health as well as the other industries that create pollutants. Health communication strategies used by the government or health communicators can also have great impacts on the health of a stakeholder. Such communication strategy may be not enough to bring about sustainability in health as long as the human right aspect is not included in the strategy. Sustainability in health will be discussed in more detail later in this chapter. In order to empower and mobilize the stakeholders to wake up on health-related issues by participating in health campaigns and changing health behavior, the critical perspective of communication within the multiplicity framework should serve this purpose. Also, the critical perspective Warren and Fassett (2011: 6-7) present can be adapted to be used in health communication for sustainability in a way that it informs us not to just understand what we experience about health, well-being, sickness and diseases within cultural contexts, but that we should bear the responsibility to question and appraise what is valuable and meaningful for us and others in our community. Through the collaborative construction and negotiation of meaning between the self and others, we can make informed choices and, in a hopeful way, we could imagine possibilities for health behavior change, growth of collaborative well-being and renewal of existing good health behaviors.

Rethinking Communication About Health

The communication that we are going to discuss in this chapter is certainly not a transmission model. A transfer of meaning through a conduit of sender-message-channel-receivers is too simplistic. A reception model of communication, which takes account of the 'power of the audience' in giving meaning to messages according to the context and the culture of receivers, should be considered (McQuail 2005: 73). That means that health communicators should keep in mind at all times that the intended message sent may be interpreted differently by audiences. The cultural context of the stakeholder shapes and defines the meaning (Warren & Fassett 2011: 7). In a critical perspective, cultural locations and communication create power. We interrogate and engage social meaning to explore how communication creates and undermines power and privilege (Warren & Fassett 2011: 13). A critical theoretical perspective is relevant to analyse power relationships in health institutions and practices; the hegemony of ideologies that back up the decision to shift the responsibility of the health care system from the state to the individual; the impact of social processes on health, ill-health states, and lifestyle choices (Foucault 1973; Hepburn 1988: 62).

In the contemporary globalization era, digital media help feed back the response of the audience or aid the interactive communication between the health communicator and the stakeholder. The boundary between the health communicators and the mass media is quite blurred due to the World Wide Web and social media networks. Each of us can be the mass media as we send and resend and create health messages and information continuously. We should bear in mind that we are communicating among groups of subcultures with unique individuals who have diverse backgrounds. Each of them is not just a silent audience; they can respond, reason logically, and express feelings and emotions. In *Chapter 4*, we learned that health inequalities can be innate and constructed by the socials. That does not mean that we have to accept these inequalities. Communication about health for sustainability should aim to reduce inequalities to live up to the declaration of universal human rights that, "all men are created equal." Not only do we need to get the message across, we need to empower and mobilize our community to rethink, participate to improve individual and community health and the environment. This leads us to the next two important discussions in this chapter: health communication for sustainability, and intercultural health communication.

COMMUNICATING ABOUT HEALTH FOR SUSTAINABLE DEVELOPMENT

Hugman and Bartolomei (2014: 21) state that development implies the capacity of people to achieve things they value in life that can be extended and enhanced. Phra Payutto (1998: 183-184), a renowned Thai Buddhist monk and philosopher, emphasizes that human development should be in line with natural environment conservation, not exploiting other humans or the environment, maintaining of self-contentment, having the wisdom to accept differences among mankind, and understanding that there are different paths to development with the aim of conserving the environment. Sustainability from Payutto's point of view can be described as a holistic view of how the physical environment is related to the social environment while realizing that each human being is an inseparable part of nature (Payutto 2006: 17-18). According to Payutto (2013), sustainability must have three dimensions: (1) the environment dimension, which has three main problems: the overpopulating rate; the depletion of natural resources; and releasing pollutants to the environment; (2) the development dimension, which includes science, technology, and economic behavior (e.g., production, consumption, and income distribution); and (3) the human development dimension. He emphasizes the human development dimension should include three aspects: (1) lifestyle and occupation, the discipline of living and working and learning how to produce, consume, share, and live in harmony with the environment; (2) mind, such as development of ethics, strength of the mind, kind-heartedness, and happiness; and (3) wisdom, meaning development of knowledge, understanding, concepts, attitude, and values. Payutto's point of view is more or less in line with the new concept, "neo-sustainability," introduced by Farley and Smith (2014). From their point of view, the broad definition of sustainable development (as in the Brundtland Report[19]) cannot set limits to the overconsumption culture that is using up our natural resources. Therefore, they came up with a new definition: "neo-sustainability.. This new definition is based on three rules:

[19] Development that meets the needs of the present without compromising the ability of future generations to meet their own needs (WCED 1987).

"1. Limits: there are natural limits to growth.
2. Environmental primacy: these limits are dictated by the environment, and therefore actions in any system must adhere to the carrying capacity of the earth's natural systems.
3. Systems thinking: because environmental, economic, and social systems are nested systems, actions must be based on systems thinking which accounts for multi-level impacts and the influences that generate impacts." (Farley & Smith 2014: 152).

In sum, sustainability requires knowledge, attitude, ethics, and behavioral change. As explained in *Chapter 1*, sustainability in health concerns social freedom, physical freedom, and inner freedom. Social freedom is an ability to be content without exploiting others, and that means respecting universal human rights as well. Rights to health also require shared organization because they go beyond the capacities of individuals (Hugman & Bartolomei 2014: 23). In the health communication realm, gender equality, rights of marginalized groups, rights of the elderly, and rights to access to primary health care should be on the top agenda. Physical freedom is freedom from want and deprivation of basic needs. This means poverty should be eradicated so that citizens of any nation could be able to fulfill their basic needs. External factors to assist are the family and community, school and mass communication, social environment including natural habitat and man-made environment, and the promotion of a positive culture. Internal factors do also rely on these external factors. However, we need to develop our inner freedom or inner peace, which is happiness based on less consumption and low resource utilization.

Health communication for sustainable development concerns the integration of five communication approaches, as presented in *Chapter 1*. They are behavior change communication, mass communication, advocacy communication, participatory communication, and communication for structural and sustainable social change. Strategies of communication can be both top-down and bottom-up models depending on the severity and contagiousness of the diseases and the context or enabling environment. Health communication in line with the multiplicity paradigm should give more weight to one of the last three approaches: advocacy, participatory, and communication for structural and sustainable social change. The rights-based approach or the critical perspective characterizes the last approach. However, mixing and matching with the first two approaches – behavioral change communication and mass communication – would work as long as the last three approaches are given priority. Let's discuss each approach in relation to health communication.

Behavioral Change Communication for Health for All

This is where personal communication comes into the picture. It can be a healthcare provider and patient interaction, or public health authority and stakeholders, or health communicator, or health volunteer and stakeholders in the community. It can also be an educator and students, or a health communicator and students, or a community leader/health professional/religious leader/news representative/ politician/practitioner/producer of popular culture/institutional representative and stakeholders. It can be discussions among students, among community dwellers, among teachers, and among family members. Communication exchange and interaction topics include, but are not limited to, what follows:

- General hygiene: how to brush teeth correctly; how to wash hands with soap correctly; how to wash fruit and vegetable correctly to reduce pesticides; how to select soap and shampoo to suit us; how to get rid of lice, etc.
- Basic sanitary: how to do housekeeping; how to do the dishes in such a way that we do not waste too much water and the dishes are clean; a comparison of seated toilets and squatting toilets (used in certain areas in developing countries), etc.
- Exercise and fitness: the usefulness of yoga; aerobic exercises like Zumba; aerobic or ballroom dancing; correct breathing exercises; tai chi; chi gong; how to check our fitness level, etc;
- Health literacy: expiry dates on canned food; food label reading and interpreting; first aids at home; toxics from medicines; how to get rid of old medicines, etc.
- Food safety: how many days a week we can eat seafood; what kind of fish or vegetable or fruit that we cannot consume in large amounts because of nitrite or mercury accumulation in the body; danger of Styrofoam food containers; toxin from peanuts; hormones and antibiotics in meat and poultry, etc.
- Nutrition: how drinking too much carbonated soft drinks affects bone density; why we should not warm certain cooked foods such as mushrooms or spinach again; what constitutes a balanced diet or the correct food pyramid; what is saturated fat; nutritious values of organic produce versus traditionally grown produce, etc.
- General clinical knowledge: how high levels of high density lipoproteins affect our health; how cholesterol, triglycerides, uric acid, glucose level, etc. affect our health.
- Environmental sustainability: biodegradable plastic; garbage separation and disposal; donation and recycling of goods; organically home-grown produce, waste water management etc.
- Disease prevention: vaccination at certain stages of our life; pasteurization; sterilization; condom use against HIV; blood screenings; herbal medicine, homeopathy etc.
- Chronic disease management: eating portion and quality of food control in case of diabetes management; types of food that should be avoided when having certain diseases such as gout or diabetes; how to exercise appropriately to the age; the importance of taking medication on time and with correct dosage; how to do the Kegel exercise in case of incontinency, how to live with your pacemaker etc.
- Health control and management, e.g., the BMI measurement, health check-ups according to age group and gender, how to manage a backache, how to prevent from choking, etc.
- Self-discipline coaching, such as no littering; no smoking in public; no coughing and sneezing without covering mouth; using a hygiene mask when having a cold, etc.

Interpersonal communication can be individual-based and group-based. Interpersonal communication can be supported with publicity media. School-based intervention falls in the group-based category. If geared towards public advocacy, interpersonal communication at all levels can be accountable for social justice in health. Public advocacy means "engaging the public through careful, thoughtful, and responsible communication toward an end that seeks a better world for our communities and our families" (Warren & Fassett 2015: 39). The main aim is to engage the patient or the stakeholder to be a "health agency," meaning that the person is empowered to take control and manage their own health and make informed choices or consent. Keep in mind that the public health services, politics, medical association and lobbyists, the Pharma-, Cosme-, and Nutri-ceutical industry, the entertainment industry, and the news industry set agendas for health research, health priorities, health services, consumption of medicine, drugs, health-related products and all these impinge on the health of an individual (Parrot 2009). Successful interpersonal communication for public advocacy at an individual- or group-base depends on knowing the audience, selecting a topic and forming a thesis, knowing how to voice, problem-posing, having reflexivity, having praxis, and critical listening (Warren & Fassett 2011: 37-45, Freire 1993). To elaborate, knowing the audience means that we should know the background of the persons we are communicating with. Audience analysis through the focus group technique is a probability sampling to find 5 to 8 people for an in-depth discussion on selected topics. Selecting the topic means developing a purpose of communication and generating a topic and forming that topic into a thesis or overarching claim to suit the interests and background of the audience. Knowing how to voice is the way health communicators feel they can effectively share their meaning and expectations with the audience. Problem-posing is a way to draw out participation and contributions from the audience. It is a way to acknowledge that the audience consists of active participants who can be empowered to start up a change process. Reflexivity is gauging one's own position, engagement, and emotion while communicating about health. Praxis is reflection and understanding that our health communication as an act has empowered the audience in critical thinking and critical engaging in health related issues. By engaging in compassionate critical listening, we could develop dialogic communication, which is the process by which the health communicator and the stakeholder(s) engage, exchange, and share or contradict meaning or interests in an ethical and respectful manner.

Interpersonal communication is important for "social support" against risk-taking behaviors. "Just say no" to drugs, tobacco, alcohol, and unsafe sex is not enough. Welch Cline (2003: 287) advised that influences of everyday communication for health:

> "(1) Are anchored more in the social reality and social norms of participants than in health knowledge, health information, and traditionally defined health beliefs and behaviors;
> (2) Are embedded in social situations that can be understood only through the realities of the participants;
> (3) May be positive or negative; and
> (4) May be planned or incidental."

Social support can be verbal and nonverbal communication that helps manage health-related uncertainty (Albrecht & Goldsmith 2003: 265). It can be all sorts of encouragement and concern; feedback on health behavior and risks; health information and modeling of health behavior; coping facilitation; provision of referrals to health professionals and lay persons; and assistance with adherence to prescribed health regimens (Albrecht & Adelman 1987; Brownell & Shumaker 1985 in Albrecht & Goldsmith 2003: 265).

Mediated-interpersonal communication is interpersonal communication that is assisted by a medium. The medium used can be the internet, radio, television, CD, DVD, or film. One of the differences between mediated interpersonal communication and mass communication is that mediated interpersonal communication needs an individual to engage the audience but mass communication needs an organization to transmit messages via the mass media (Turow 2014: 7). This leads us to the next topic.

Mass Communication for Health for All

Mass communication as defined by Turow (2014: 9) is the industrialized production and multiple distributions of messages through technological devices. Mass communication was formerly referred to as one-way communication where a mass media organization, such as a television station, a radio station, a newspaper, a magazine, a journal, etc., sends news and information en masse. That was the assumption in the past! In the contemporary globalization period, new media technologies have characterized the postmodern culture by increasing the flow, the speed, the volume of information, the system upgradability, and interconnectivity as well as diversifying communication channels and increasing the content control by users while reducing the cost and distant sensitivity of moving information (Neuman 1991: 53-71). The increase of interactivity between the mass media organization and receivers via the mass media has made two-way communication possible. Moreover, the popularity of the social media has made an individual a mass communicator who sends and resends messages. The formerly passive mass audiences are now able to upload their still images and video clips taken by a webcam or a smartphone or a digital camera, write a blog, or post a text message on any social media network. The other receivers can give feedback and share or repost the same video clips, images, and texts to others via the network. That has made the mode of communication shift from a two-way street to multiple nodes of interactivity, thanks to smart phones, iPods, iPads, laptops, and other telecommunication applications. Nowadays, different mass media have the ability to interact with one another and that's what we call the mass media convergence (Turow 2014: 13). For instance, a newspaper can have its digital television channel, an Instagram page, a Facebook page, and a website which allows the audience to watch video clips or listen to the digital audio files. Moreover, the newspaper agency can tweet its news via Twitter. With high speed broadband internet, the audience is now able to download video clips and/or audio files from the website of the news agency. The audience can hook up a laptop with the digital TV set and watches news from the website on TV and download a series of audio files from the internet that the news agency releases (the so-called "pod cast") regularly and listen to them via an iPod or a laptop. These different media formats shape the content, especially the depth of the information. For instance, Twitter allows a limited number of 140 characters; messages sent via Twitter must be concise and straight to the point.

Nowadays the term 'network society' or 'knowledge society' is replacing the old term 'information society' as we have overloaded information in cyberspace but only some of that information can be digested and turned into knowledge. Therefore, a knowledge society has a connotation to a society wherein active information seekers live. The interconnectedness or networking indicates the high degree of interdependence in the contemporary globalization period (McQuail 2005: 106). This indicates that the audiences are no longer empty vessels but are connected to one another in the cyber web.

In the past, it was said that the mass media can trigger only the awareness of the faceless receivers and shift attention towards long-term change and "towards collective phenomena such as climates of opinion, structures of belief, definitions of reality, ideologies, cultural patterns, and institutional forms of media provision" (McQuail 2005: 460) rather than altering their attitude or change their behavior. In the Internet era, the new media can have more impact on the attitude and informed choices of the health information seekers. In Internet and healthcare studies, online information seekers become more informed about health, and sociological research has shown that accessed information serves to modify (if not evade) individual responsibility and promotes the individual expression of a personal experience of health and illness (Kivits 2013: 222-223). Active participants can get involved in the health content control or content amplification of new media. However, they can also send hyper-reality images or fake information on treatments, health experiences, herbal medicines, disease prevention online as well. This leads to the requirement of health communicators to be versed in media literacy, which will be discussed in detail in *Chapter 6*.

However, carefully geared and planned, the mass media convergence and social media can be used to inform and empower the audience by way of participatory social marketing. Let's discuss social marketing first. Social marketing is an adoption of marketing strategies selling commercial products. The same process of 4 Ps (product, pricing, place, and promotion) has been adapted to influence and inform the public on health problems such as heart infarct, high blood pressure, using condoms to prevent HIV, wearing a seat belt while driving, etc. Traditional social marketing falls into the category of the modernization paradigm, using Persuasion Theory, Behavioral Theory, and the Transtheoretical model. More modern is the Social Media Marketing (SMM) model. SMM, according to Barker, Barker, Bormann, and Neher (2013: 3) is:

> "A term that describes use of social networks, online communities, blogs, wikis or any other online collaborative media for marketing, sales, public relations and customer service. Common social media marketing tools include Twitter, blogs, LinkedIn, Facebook, Flickr and YouTube."

According to Barker et al. (2013: 3), SMM is different from traditional marketing because it does not need the place and promotion to dissipate new ideas. The social interconnectedness and online conversations will spread the words or buzz or newsworthy events, videos, tweets, or blog entries. It is more than a two-way street of social marketing in a sense that it initiates and encourages participation and dialogue. The idea of SMM can be used to promote health. Instead of the traditional social marketing, we can call this new way, "Social Media for Social Marketing," or SMSM. This gives way to a new opportunity to initiate "participatory social marketing" which consists of participatory SMSM (online) and offline participatory marketing campaigns for health for all.

Participatory social marketing can be categorized within the multiplicity paradigm using the Self Determination Theory, the Behavior Development and Change Model, and the Social Networks and Social Support model. Traditional social marketing uses a strategy of market segmentation to specify customer profiles; audience analysis by using a focus group; identifying the objectives of targeted behavior changes, tailoring communication or personalizing the message, and adapting strategies such as branding to educate and promote the adoption, maintenance of health behaviors; and prevention of health risk-taking behaviors (British Medical Journal 2006). As smart phones and digital cameras are now affordable, social marketing on health behavior can be done via social media and media production can be participatory, as defined in the UNESCO report on self-management, access, and participation (Berrigan 1979: 8), that stakeholders and media producers can take part in the research, production and self-management of the media. For instance, senior students at a high school would like to produce a social media marketing film. They announce this idea via the school website and social media. A group of volunteers meets to debate on which topic to choose. For instance, a campaign against smoking is selected. By making decisions together as to who needs to do what, this process is participatory. This campaign will be designed and operated by the students and volunteer teachers. By participation, data gathering through in-depth interviews of students who smoke, who do not smoke, and who quit smoking can be done by volunteer students. More interviews can be conducted with teachers, the parents of the students, the classmates and close friends of the students. Script writing can be done through brain-storming. Filming and editing can be done by a group of volunteers using a digital video camera and a FinalCutPro editing program. Students can produce a short film showing the circumstances in which a student can quit smoking and upload it on the school website and social media network. By teaching how anyone can build up autonomy or intrinsic motivation not to smoke, the video would build empathy to those who smoke, ways to assess health risks from smoking, and provide activities to substitute smoking. Next, the video would encourage competency by not making harsh criticism on those who smoke but provide concerns, positive thinking, and respect for them. These ideas are based on the SDT theory. By setting up a social support discussion page for people who want to quit smoking on the school website and announce it on the video, peer-to-peer help is becoming instrumental in changing behavior. A teacher can help coach life skills training on the video as well.

Under the multiplicity paradigm, participatory social marketing can be summarized as follows.

1) Participatory setting of objectives and budget. Together the producers lay down objectives and set goals; how to reach those goals within the permitted budget.
2) Participatory selection of a social media platform and study the demographics of the users in the community that prefer the selected social media platforms.
3) Participatory design of a storyboard, production timeline, production task assignment.
4) Participatory selection of ways to the publicity of the product. Interpersonal communication can be used. See details about other media in *Chapter 6*.

Advocacy Communication for Health for All

The World Health Organization (WHO) uses advocacy health communication to enhance knowledge of diseases among the public and people living with the disease and empower them to express their needs and take action. Mass media can play two kinds of health advocacy: (a) supporting health promotion or disease prevention by disseminating messages that encourage the public to support the projects; and (b) providing the decision-makers with the necessary information and feedback needed to reach a decision on health (Servaes & Malikhao 2010: 43). Advocacy communication means using two-way communication to influence key decision makers to support policy changes in local, national and international policy discussions and to sustain accountability and commitment from governmental and international actors (WHO 2015d).

For sustainability, advocacy communication should be modified to fit in the multiplicity paradigm by adding the participatory aspect to it. Participatory-based advocacy communication is a communication strategy which empowers the grassroots and lets their voice be heard. This strategy will focus on listening and cooperation rather than on 'telling what to do.' Therefore, health advocacy is comprised of social support and empowerment strategies (Servaes & Malikhao 2010: 43).

Important criteria for the success of advocacy messages are relevance, timing, validity, cultural sensitivity, orientation of the relevant stakeholder groups, planning, communication, and dissemination of information (Servaes & Malikhao 2010: 48). To elaborate, the health issue has to be considered relevant to the several stakeholder groups. It has to be put on the agenda at the right time. The information and statistics provided have to be valid and meaningful. The information about health or diseases should be tailored to the audiences and be in line with the understandings and expectations of people or stakeholders. Stakeholder groups have to be trained in interpreting data, so that they are able to understand them.

Participatory Communication for Health for All

Participation is a means to achieve the objectives of the community members in developing their lives and it is also an end or a core aspect of what is necessary to live a decent life (Hugman & Bartolomei 2014: 19). Participatory communication encompasses the cultural identity of local communities and of democratization at the individual and local, national, and international levels (Servaes & Malikhao 2008: 169). It is a strategy which emphasizes interpersonal communication and multi-community media. Participation of the grassroots, which indicates the direction of a bottom-up approach, is not only a challenge to the top-down power of the empiricist-and-dominant modernization paradigm, but is also a challenge to the universal concept of the "right-to-communicate" without considering the diversity and pluralism of the stakeholders (Huesca 2008: 188-189). Therefore, under the framework of the multiplicity paradigm, participatory health communication is not a camouflage of a diffusion theory or a two-step flow of information, which stipulates that there are steps of progress starting from hearing innovations in health-related areas to favorable attitude towards the innovation aided by mass communication and up to the ultimate level of adoption of that innovation and finally change risk-taking behavior to a favorable health behavior aided by opinion leaders through interpersonal communication. Rather, participatory health communication aims at redistributing power among the public health policy-makers and top public health authority to the stakeholders by ways of developing the capacity of community action for health literacy, community health and disease prevention, and environmental health in a given community. Community media (either Websites, community radio, community TV, community theaters, community exhibitions and fairs, etc.) as well as selected social media can be the channels to arouse the community interests and participation in health-related issues. The most important aspects of participatory communication are that the diversity, pluralism, and human rights have to be taken into account (Huesca 2008: 193). Social justice, human rights, and virtues are the ethical criteria to examine participation for health in the community. Hugman and Bartolomei (2014: 20) explain that social justice means fairness or balance to be achieved between competing interests; rights are about what it is to be human; and virtues are about the way in which the character of a person might be directed towards human flourishing, for both that person and others.

Communication for Structural and Sustainable Social Change for Health for All

This is the ultimate level of health communication for sustainable development. This is not a utopian approach. It can be used if health communicators include their roots, i.e., their communities up to the national level, diverse cultures and ethnicity, and diverse health practices, and human rights, especially the rights to an appropriate environment and access to an appropriate healthcare system, into the development of an indigenous health policy, health communication strategies, and assessment. A combination of all the afore-mentioned communication approaches can be used to empower the stakeholders to act for the uplifting and sustaining of their community on health and media literacy, right information on health and disease prevention, environmental health, health behavior and access to affordable and quality health care system.

I would like to connect Kennedy's (2008: 151-166) discussion on attitudes and roles of development field workers with the attitudes and roles needed for health communicators for sustainable development. As stated in *Chapter 1* human development must come first. A health communicator is a person who is capable of transgressing the attitude of pity to sympathy and, finally, to empathy. This is not a kind of diffusion of innovations to develop steps to adopt empathy while using media. The inner self can be polished, tamed, and molded from experiences gained in the health communication field. More importantly, this process of self-development can be trained and taught.

- *Pity* is a condescending or paternalistic attitude to help stakeholders; a pitiful health communicator is detached in his expression of emotions and shares only 'expert-advice' with the stakeholders (Kennedy 2008: 151). Its connotation is a top-down approach of health communication that feeds health information or health aids to the community like pouring water into an empty vessel. The role of the health communicator is a health broker. This is an analogy to a social broker who serves as a go-between, gatekeeping the information flow between communities or groups and government decision-makers (Kennedy: 154). As a go-between, the health communicator takes the health literacy and health information of the stakeholders in his/her hands as well as the expectation of efficiency from the government.
- *Sympathy* is feeling sorry for the distress of stakeholders and willing to be more involved in the action of helping out but not having enough time to engage time, energy, and interest to assist the stakeholders. "Sympathy connotes a spontaneous emotion rather than a considered attitude," states Kennedy (2008: 152). A

sympathetic health communicator works as a health advocate. Kennedy (2008: 155) defines the social advocate as a development field worker who acts on behalf of the community or group s/he represents. The health advocate represents the stakeholders to raise their voice to the authority on health issues. However, in the long run this process is not sustainable. The explanation is that when the health advocate cannot live up to the expectations of the stakeholders, anger and frustration will ensue. Thus, health advocacy is a short-term solution to the health issues of a community.

- *Empathy* is the ultimate attitude that can be developed for sustainability in health communication. According to Kennedy (2008: 153), empathy…

"… goes beyond sympathy and is characterized by a conscious involvement with a person's situation, in the sense of vicarious identification. Empathy implies a willingness to take the time to learn and understand how the other person perceives a person, place, or situation. The empathic individual is willing to become vulnerable to the other person be being involved in an open-ended relationship on the other person's terms."

An empathetic communicator acts as a *social mobilizer*. A social mobilizer believes in the collective power of the stakeholders who can act together to build up their own capacity on identifying their own needs, arriving at a consensus for action, and taking their own direct action (Kennedy 2008:158). By analogy, an empathetic health communicator who acts as a health mobilizer puts strong beliefs in the capability of the community members to plan and implement their own health literacy, health campaigns, and any change process regarding health and environment in the community.

Sustainable development on health should be defined as the process of social mobilization empowered by stakeholders, some of whom act as health communicators, and empathetic health communicators from outside the community, for the goals of (1) achieving and maintaining health literacy and media literacy for the people in the community, so that the people make informed choices on issues related to individual health and healthcare; (2) achieving and maintaining community capacity and networking with other communities to problem solving on community health, for social justice in health and collective well-being, and disease prevention, and to advocate knowledge, attitude, worldview, value, behavioral and structural change for a collective healthy lifestyle and human-friendly environment.

The following criteria to assess whether a health communication project is in support of sustainable development or not, are adapted from Servaes et al. (2012: 12-17):

1) *Actors*. That includes international and local NGOs, government, private providers of health services, and local community members which may include opinion leaders, community activists, tribal elders, youth, etc. A sustainability indicator should be whether the local community members are involved in the discussion and assessment of the health project, or not.
2) *Factors*: can be structural or conjectural. A structural factor is the economic one. Who pays for the up and running of the project? The social factor in terms of whose benefits should be taken into account. Sustainability depends on whether both budgets and labor-capital relationships are included, or not.
3) *Levels*. At which level is the project aimed at: community, regional, state or the local unit, local municipality, or metropolis municipality, or government. Sustainability

depends on whether a locally-based and specific project is preferred more than a large scale project, or not.

4) *Types of communication.* Is it a combination of participation, advocacy, mass media/new media, and interpersonal communication under the framework of the multiplicity paradigm, or not?
5) *Communication channels,* for instance, radio, ICT, TV, print, online digital media, etc., and cost effectiveness of choosing the channels should be taken into consideration. The communication channels chosen should be compatible with the actors, and affordable.
6) *Messages* refer to the content of a project or campaign; whether the message is developed by and for the community, or not.
7) *Process of communication.* If it is a sustainable one, it should be interactive, dialogical or at least two-way communication.
8) *Methods.* A mixed method of quantitative and qualitative techniques is a good indicator of sustainability for a deeper understanding of not only the epidemiological status but also the impacts and concerns of the locals. The qualitative method, which assesses the political, social and cultural infrastructures, should not be overlooked.
9) *The clarity, reception, and production of the message.* This needs a good understanding of intercultural communication, as will be discussed next.

Health communication from a critical perspective for sustainable development should be on the premises that human rights are respected; social justice is achieved; and virtues are met. Participation is a way to achieve human rights and is in itself to be a right. In order to achieve social justice, rights, and virtues, it is important to communicate across cultural and subcultural contexts of gender, age, social status, education, religious groups, beliefs, and with marginalized groups to encourage participation, advocate for change, and mobilize the community. This leads to our next topic.

INTERCULTURAL COMMUNICATION ABOUT HEALTH

Stiff with conceit
we make no real contact
believing so much
in our opinions and desires
the links we seem to create
are merely apparent
Jayasaro Bhikku (Ajahn Jayasaro) (2012: 108)

Intercultural communication about health is not only interpersonal communication of healthcare providers and patients. It can be group-, community-, or organization-based. Any social mobilizer who wants to initiate participatory advocacy communication and communication for empowerment on a health project needs to possess intercultural skills. Intercultural communication concerns the sharing of information for mutual understanding and agreeable identity. Identity has many types depending on the social contexts and time:

sexual, gender, political, religious, etc. From the definitions of culture described in *Chapter 4*, it is important to state again that culture is socially constructed and subjective.

Edward Hall (1959) introduced the concept of *cultural relativity*. It is based on the assumption that there are no superior cultures, and culture, though it has its own strengths and weaknesses, should not be compared in terms of values or merits (Hall 1959). Not only does intercultural communication concern national cultures, it also concerns the studies of the subcultures classified by tribes, communities, classes, and ethnic groups (Geertz 1995). Intercultural skills on health issues are the competency to communicate with subculture groups about health issues with the knowledge that there are health inequalities caused by the dynamic interaction of determinants.

To be competent in intercultural communication, one should understand the four building blocks of it: culture, communication, context, and power (Martin & Nakayama 2014: 64). Culture is learned, shared, and expressed (Martin and Nakayama 2014: 64). Communication is a sharing process of meaning. Through the communication process not only do we transmit information and knowledge, we also construct our own meaning and share, extend, create, and preserve collective memory. We, thus, maintain and create a sense of community (Uzelac 2008: 10). The belief that community, culture and health are related to one another has been here since the ancient time (MacLachlan 1997: 32). Context is the social setting in which communication takes place. Power is hidden in the way social institutions communicate. Power is the ability to make others do what one wants. It is hidden in the way we communicate: verbally and nonverbally. Successful intercultural communicators should observe and reflect upon the way they communicate. They avoid ethnocentrism, stereotyping, prejudice, and discrimination imbedded in the way they communicate, because that would destroy the communication process.

Ethnocentrism is the belief that one's own cultural group is superior to all other cultural groups (Martin & Nakayama 2014: 55). It is learned through a socialization process, but it can be unlearned by anthropological training. Meeting people from different cultures and learn to appreciate other cultures, stepping out of one's own culture and be in a different culture for a while, will help the reflexivity of a communicator.

Stereotypes are ways of generalizing a group of people and judging a person on this basis. Stereotyping in the health related field is, for instance, the argument that HIV/AIDS is caused by gay people, or people living with HIV/AIDS are sinful people. Martin and Nakayama (2014: 59) advise how to get rid of stereotypes by (1) recognizing the negative stereotypes that we all possess, and (2) obtaining individual information that can counteract the stereotype.

Prejudice is a negative attitude toward a cultural group and that may arise from a personal need to feel positive about one's own group and negative about others, or from perceived or real threats (Martin & Nakayama 2014: 59). This subconscious attitude can be undone by training to appreciate other cultures.

Discrimination is a behavior resulting from stereotyping or prejudice (Martin & Nakayama 2014: 62). Martin and Nakayama (2014: 62) state that the power plus prejudice equals "ism"; be it sexism, racism, ageism, elitism. Discrimination can be interpersonal, collective, and/or institutional:

> "Discrimination may range from very subtle nonverbal (lack of eye contact, exclusion of someone from a conversation), to verbal insults and exclusion from job or

other economic opportunities, to physical violence and systematic elimination of the group, or genocide" (Martin & Nakayama 2014: 62).

It would be ridiculous if a social mobilizer for health or a social advocate for change in a health related area discriminates against others. Discrimination can be unlearned by practicing one's mind to have empathy and compassion to others who are from a different culture. Discrimination may come from a religious belief but mostly comes from the upbringing and socialization process. According to Payutto (2007: 55-63), as stated in *Chapter 1*, one of the beliefs or ditthi that held control of world civilization is the perception that fellow human beings are not "fellow human beings." This perception has been the foundation of the aforementioned barriers (ethnocentrism, stereotyping, prejudice, and discrimination) in the history of mankind. A well-educated person is the person who can eradicate these negative values from his or her sub-consciousness. In other words, the educated ones are the ones who can polish their egos and have good human relations along with being competent and knowledgeable in the field. To polish one's ego can start from practicing to rejoice with others' success, learning to understand others from others' perspectives, sympathizing with others who are less fortunate and practicing equanimity of the mind.

A human rights approach is the way to fight against discrimination. Rights of children and women should be advocated as well as the rights of ethnic minorities and LGBT. Everyone, including animals, has a right to be treated fairly, kindly, and respectfully. Education is the key to promote a right-based approach to health communication.

Here are some tips on intercultural communication to empower health behaviors as adapted from Martin and Nakayama's (2010: 381-392) report: person-contextual dialectic; differences-similarities dialectic; cultural-individual dialectic; and privilege-disadvantage dialectic.

- *Person-contextual dialectic*: Health communicators should be able to differentiate types of meaning of words: denotative, connotative, contextual, and figurative. Kim (2012: 50-52) explains that denotative is a simple relationship between the words and the corresponding objects or action (e.g., mother); connotative meaning is the evaluative, emotional, affective meaning of the word (i.e., a person can be differently described as strong-willed or pig-headed); contextual meaning is how words can change their meaning depending upon the context (i.e., racing horses can actually mean horses for racing or meaning the way people are competing like race horses); figurative meaning is the difficulty across cultural health communicator encounters while trying to understand figurative idioms used in another language (i.e., an English speaking person may say "it's Greek to me!" while a French speaking person may refer to it as, "it's Chinese to me!").

  Also critical reading should be emphasized. When reading, one must pay attention to how the writer describes what is going on; how the writer indicates attitude to self, subject, and reader; and how the content of the text is organized (Fairclough 1992: 93).

  Health communicators should be able to differentiate personal health behaviors, which are consistent from situation to situation (such as washing hands after using the bathroom or brushing teeth at least two times a day, or covering one's mouth while sneezing, or coughing), and some behaviors that are influenced by social contexts or social networks (such as binge drinking, smoking, sharing syringes among injection drug users, or using condoms).

- *Differences-similarities dialectic*: communication structures can be high-context and low-context in culture; direct and indirect presentation culture; and conflict avoidance culture. According to Hall (1976: 91) high –context communication or messages can be found in countries like Japan, China, and Korea. That means communication depends on figurative and approximate language; sees tasks as a function of the relationship; prefers indirect style in writing and speaking; expects decision making within the relationship; relies on nonverbal communication; respects and utilizes silence; and subordinates use of detailed information. A low-context culture can be found in countries like Switzerland (German speaking part), Germany, Scandinavia, and the US. They believe in explicit (literal) communication; keep job tasks separate from relationships; use direct style in writing and speaking; value individual initiative and decision making; rely on verbal communication; become uncomfortable with silence, and present facts, statistics, and other details (Kim 2012: 69 adapted from Sherron & Deborah 1997).

  Health communicators should be able to address both differences and similarities of the community or a person they work with to that of their own. People from a different culture may have different ways to express pains, or select treatment, or need their own rituals for healing. Non-verbal communication may be different as well. In Thailand people avoid eye contact as it is considered polite and respectful not to look straight into the eyes of a senior person, while people in the West must look straight into the eyes of the counterpart to express sincerity. A reminder for health communicators is always to have a non-judgmental attitude. We all have at least one similarity: we love to live a healthy life. If we could see others as other human beings who need love, compassion and understanding, and avoid pains just like us, we would treat others with respect and kindness. Sharing and caring should be the starting point for a good health communicator.
- *Cultural-individual dialectic*: the cultural context in which we are communicating about health should be understood. It is important that a social mobilizer checks the values, worldview and symbolic interactions of that particular culture or subculture by interviewing or talking with the people, or having a focus group discussion, or reading from records and documents about that particular culture. The ability of a social mobilizer to speak the local language or dialect is a plus. If a social mobilizer or a media advocate does not speak the language or dialect, a good interpreter, whom many people in the community know, should earn the mobilizer some trust to begin with. Galanti (2008: 2) suggests that health communicators should understand their own culture and biases, be sensitive to other people's cultures, and appreciate the differences. In *Chapter 4*, I also identified 'respect other people's culture' as a good way to communicate on health in any cultural context. However, we have to admit that there are certain cultural norms that hinder the sustainability of health such as sharing one's wife with guests or polygamous behavior (anarchists may call this behavior polyamory). These behaviors would sustain the spread of HIV/AIDS. Another example is the genital mutilation of young girls in certain cultures. The girls are at risk of infection, but – more importantly – it is against their human right. It is

as gender-biased as the extinctive culture of binding feet for women in traditional Chinese culture before the Cultural Revolution.

One of the main cultural value dimensions, Hofstede (2001) identifies, is the difference between collectivism versus individualism. Countries such as China, Venezuela, Colombia, Indonesia, and Korea tend to be more collectivistic, while Western countries such as the US, Germany, and Australia tend to be more individualistic. The collectivists stress harmony in interpersonal relationships. They do not join many groups. Group harmony and achievement is more important than those of the individual. Age or seniority is cherished. Members of the group prefer interdependence and consider individual aggressive behavior negative. The individualists tend to join many groups. Achievement of an individual is highly prized. Status differences are rejected. Democracy is emphasized. Members tend to be remote and distant. Personal independence is cherished.

- *Privilege-disadvantage dialectic*: this is about power and power differentials in intercultural relationships. A low power distance society is a society that accepts power relations in a more democratic manner (such as in Western cultures), while a high power distance society is a society where relations are more autocratic or paternalistic (such as in Asian cultures). The masculinity and femininity of a culture also manifests power differentials. Hofstede (2001: 50) explains that feminine cultures have the following characteristics: caring for others is a dominant value; focused on relationships; cherishing modesty; working to live; managing aims for consensus; emphasizing equality, solidarity, and quality; and solving conflicts by compromise. Masculine cultures emphasize material success as a dominant value; possessions; assertiveness of men; living to work; managing with decisive fashion; competition and performance; and fighting out to solve conflicts.

  Regarding communicating about health, health communicators may be simultaneously privileged and disadvantaged. Privileged in a sense that they have good connections with community leaders; they may already know the strength and weakness of the community regarding health and well-being. Disadvantaged in the sense that they may find resistance from a group of people in the community; they may need to assess the situation. Relationship building is important. According to Hofstede (2001: 125), relationships are both static and dynamic. Southeast Asian countries have weaker uncertainty avoidance. That means they are comfortable in ambiguous situations. They do not need more rules. They are more tolerant of innovative ideas and motivated by achievement. For Western countries, uncertainty is a threat. People fear ambiguous situations. They need rules. They are resistant to innovation and are motivated by security.

  Health communicators should understand that empowerment does not happen in a short period of time. It takes time to mobilize people to take health issues in their hands. Media advocacy such as edutainment can help spread dialogues on health related issues.

- *History/Past-Present/Future Dialectic*: it is always useful to research the history of health issues in a community in order to understand the current situation and to plan for the future. The level of analysis can be individual, family, ethnic group, community, institution, or a nation.

Health communication is not limited to only patient and healthcare provider communication. It is about the communication between or among an observable unit (individual/group of people or virtual group/community/organization/nation) to achieve health awareness, attitude, and behavior, either through the mass media, or the new media, or through human communication.

In order to sustain the level of wellness, health communicators need good cultural competencies. A critical perspective of language in intercultural communication should be included.

CONCLUSION

Communication for/about health requires interdisciplinary knowledge. As communication for sustainability approaches were explained, it should now be clear that a successful health communicator for sustainable development should be a health advocate or a health mobilizer. In order to achieve this, communication skills must be trained. Writing professionally, speaking with loving kindness and compassion, listening carefully, and having good human relation skills are important to build up mutual trust and collaboration. Human relation skills include intercultural communication skills to connect with everyone. More importantly, a health communicator must have a sense of humor. Being flexible and being able to respond, not to react immediately, needs to be learned. Keeping composure and professionalism is an essential skill. Moreover, a successful health communicator must possess basic computer skills and proficiency with search engines to navigate the Internet. Knowledge of coding or graphic design would help in case one needs to design or master a website. This leads us to discuss choices of tools or media in the next chapter.

REFERENCES

Albrecht, T. L. & Adelmen, M. B. (1987). *Communicating Social Support*. Newbury Park, CA: Sage.

Albrecht, T. L. & Goldsmith, D. J. (2003). Social Support, Social Networks, and Health. In T. L. Thompson, A. Dorsey, K. I. Miller, R. Parrott (Eds.) *Handbook of Health Communication*. New York-London: Lawrence Erlbaum Associates., pp. 263-284.

Berrigan, F. J. (1979). *Community Communications. The Role of Community Media in Development.* Paris: UNESCO.

Boyd-Barrett, O. (2015). *Media Imperialism*. Los Angeles-London-New Dehli-Singapore-Washington DC: SAGE Publications Inc.

Brown, A. (1995). *Organisational Culture*. London: Pitman Publishing.

Brownell, A. & Shumaker, S. A. (1985). Where Do We Go from Here? The Policy Implications of Social Support. *Journal of Social Issues*, 41, 111-121.

Carey, J. W. (1992). *Communication as Culture: Essays on Media and Society*. New York-London: Routledge.

Evans, D. (2006). How Social Marketing Works in Healthcare. *British Medical Journal*. May 20. 332(7551) pp. 1207-1210. (Doi: 10.1136/bmj.332.7551.1207-a.

Fairclough, N. (1992). *Critical Language Awareness*. New York: Longman.

Farley, H. M. & Smith, Z. A. (2014). *Sustainability. If It's Everything, Is It Nothing?* London-New York: Routledge.

Foucault, M. (1973). *The Birth of the Clinic*. London: Tavistock.

Fox, E. (2012). Rethinking Health Communication in Aid and Development. In R. Obregon & S. Waisbord (Eds.) *The Handbook of Global Health Communication*. West Sussex: Wiley-Blackwell, a John Wiley & Sons, Ltd., Publication, pp. 52-69.

Freire, P. (1993). *Education for Critical Consciousness*. New York: Continuum.

Galanti, G. (2008). *Caring for Patients from Different Cultures* (4th ed.). Philadelphia, PA: University of Pennsylvania Press.

Geertz, C. (1995). *After the Fact: Two Countries, four decades, one anthropologist*. Cambridge, MA: Harvard University Press.

Hall, E. T. (1959). *The Silent Language*. New York: Doubleday.

Hepburn, S. J. (1988). Western Minds, Foreign Bodies. *Medical Anthropology Quarterly* 2, pp. 59-74.

Huesca, R. (2008). Tracing the History of Participatory Communication Approaches to Development: A Critical Appraisal. In (J. Servaes ed.)*Communication for Development and Social Change*. Los Angeles: Sage.

Hofstede, G. (2001). *Culture's Consequences: Comparing Values, Behaviours, Institutions and Organizations across Nations* (2nd ed). Beverly Hills, CA: Sage Publications, Inc. (https://ad34c3acb3d2700a49a406cdff75053dd1fd8d65.googledrive.com/host/0B7aKRMPHsA89MmJrLTlRcFNSZG8/Seen%20in%20Their%20True%20Light%20(2012-05).pdf, accessed on June 26th, 2015).

Hugman, R. & Bartolomei, L. (2014). The Ethics of Participation in Community Work Practice. In A. K. Larsen, V. Sewpaul & G. O. Hole (Eds.) *Participation in Community Work. International Perspectives*. London and New York: Routledge, pp. 19-29.

Jayasaro Bhikku (2012). *Seen in their true light*. Bangkok: Panyaprateep Foundation (www.panyaprateep.org).

Kennedy, T. (2008). *Where the Rivers Meet the Sky. A Collaborative Approach to Participatory Development*. Penang, Malaysia: Southbound.

Kim, Y. M. (2012). *Critical Intercultural Communication Strategies in the Age of Glocalism*. Korea: Han Gukmoonhwasa.

Lie, R. (2003). *Spaces of Intercultural Communication: An Interdisciplinary Introduction to Communication, Culture, and Globalizing/Localizing Identities*. New Jersey: Hampton Press, Inc.

MacLachlan, M. (1997). *Culture and Health*. New York: John Wiley & Sons.

Martin, J. N. & Nakayama, T. K. (2010). *Intercultural Communication in Contexts* (5th ed.) New York: McGraw-Hill.

Martin, J. N. & Nakayama, T. K. (2014). *Experiencing Intercultural Communication. An Introduction*. New York: McGraw-Hill.

McQuail, D. (2005). *McQuail's Mass Communication Theory* (5th ed.) London-Thousand Oaks-New Delhi: Sage Publications.

Mohammed, S. N. (2011). *Communication and the Globalization of Culture*. Lanham-Boulder-New York-Toronto-Plymouth,UK: Lexington Books.

Neuman, W. R. (1991). *The Future of the Mass Audience*. Cambridge, U.K: Cambridge University Press.

Parrot, R. (2009). *Talking about Health. Why Communication Matters*. Malden, M.A: Wiley-Blackwell.

Payutto, P. A. (1998). *Sustainable Development* (3rd ed.). Bangkok: Buddhatham Foundation.

Payutto, P.A. (2006). *Sukhapava Ong Ruam Naew Buddha (Holistic well-being the Buddhist Way)*. (http://www.fungdham.com/download/book/payutto/490109-sukhapava.pdf).

Payutto, P.A. (2007). *A Buddhist Solution for the Twenty-first Century* (17th ed.) Bangkok: Pimsuay Printing.

Payutto, P.A. (2013). *Sustainable Development* (13th ed.) Bangkok: Komol Keemthong Foundation.

Servaes, J. & Malikhao, P. (2008). Development Communication Approaches in an International Perspective. In J. Servaes (Ed.) *Communication for Development and Social Change*. Los Angeles: Sage, pp. 158-179.

Servaes, J. & Malikhao, P. (2010). Advocacy Strategies for Health Communication. *Public Relations Review*, pp. 42-49. (Doi: 10.1016/j.pubrev.2009.08.017).

Servaes, J., Polk, E., Shi, S., Reilly, D. & Yukupitijage, T. (2012). Towards a Framework of Sustainability Indicators for 'Communication for Development and Social Change' Projects. *The International Communication Gazette,* pp. 1-25. (Doi: 10.1177/1748048511432598).

Sheron, B. K. & Deborah, V. (1997). *Crosstalk: Communicating in a Multicultural Workplace*. Upper Saddle River, NJ: Prentice Hall.

Thompson, J. (1995). *The Media and Modernity. A Social Theory of the Media.* Cambridge: Polity Press.

Turow, J. (2014). *Media Today. Mass Communication in a Converging World* (5th ed.) New York: Routledge.

Uzelac, A. (2008). How to Understand Digital Culture: Digital Culture—a Resource for a Knowledge Society? In A. Uzelac & B. Cvjeticanin (Eds.) *Digital Culture: The - Changing Dynamics. Zagreb, Croatia*: Institute for International Relations., pp. 7-21.

Warren, J. T. & Fassett, D. L. (2011). *Communication. A Critical/Cultural Introduction.* Los Angeles-London-New Delhi-Singapore-Washington DC: Sage Publications, Inc.

Welch Cline, R. J. (2003). Everyday Interpersonal Communication and Health. In T. L. Thompson, A. Dorsey, K. I. Miller, R. Parrott (Eds.) *Handbook of Health Communication*. New York-London: Lawrence Erlbaum Associates., pp.285-313.

Websites

World Health Organization

WHO 2015 d

http://www.who.int/tb/people_and_communities/advocacy_communication/en/, accessed October 22nd, 2015.

Chapter 6

OLD AND NEW MEDIA IN HEALTH COMMUNICATION FOR SUSTAINABLE DEVELOPMENT

ABSTRACT

This chapter discusses what constitutes traditional or old media and new media. Interactions of users with new media as a new form of mass-self communication, and the integrated impacts of digitized and traditional media on culture, called mediatization, will be explained. With increasing new media usage in our daily life, it is important that health communicators are media literates. Media literacy is defined and explained. Community media, which consist of both old and new media, as tools of communication for/about health, are the highlight of this chapter. They can be strategically integrated and planned for participatory-based health advocacy and health mobilization for improvements on healthcare policy and living conditions of members in communities.

Keywords: traditional media, hybrid media, new media, media convergence, mainstream media, alternative media, indymedia, media literacy, community media, health mobilizers, health advocates

INTRODUCTION

A picture tells a thousand words. A film tells more than a picture. Health communicators cannot claim that they are only academicians, and therefore, do not need to know about any hands-on subjects, such as basic photography, basic desktop-publishing skills, basic digital storytelling skills, etc. In the field of health communication, one needs to be well-rounded and self-reliant while economizing on resources. If a health communicator is trained to be acquainted with internet studies and basic media production, that person can empower or mobilize the stakeholders to participate in presenting on health or environmental issues with relevant images, sounds, and texts. That's why media skills and media literacy are very important assets for anybody in health communication.

Communicating for/about health and the environment requires a good media selection. Although the media do not equate the message, we should not overlook the importance of using communication technologies together with personal media to get our health-related messages across. The increase of digitized media allows for global localization, which means that the grassroots can now voice their concerns and solutions regarding community health and well-being, and environmental health. These concerns can be sent upward to the policy makers. This is a revolution! Grassroots globalization has begun.

Health knowledge sharing and access is a new way to closing the inequality gap on primary healthcare, nutrition, health literacy, first-aids, and disease prevention. Environmental health knowledge sharing and access, and surveillance of environment within the community will become more effective with the aid of digital media use and World Wide Web connections. Citizen journalists can now report wrongdoing about the environment that affects the health of the community. These types of media create a civic communication or a public sphere in which the public can take part in the discussion and decision-making that will affect their living conditions and health.

Types of Media

Media are all around us and appear in a variety of formats: news media such as print, photography, etc.; broadcast media such as radio, television, podcast, internet radio, internet television, etc.; personal media such as laptops, desktops, cell phones, smart phones (for interpersonal communication), etc.; mass media such as smart phones, billboards, T-shirts, banners, video games, etc.

We can categorize media into three types: traditional media, hybrid media, and new media. The *traditional media* or old media are those classic print media, such as books, photographs, newspaper, and magazines; electronic media such as radio and television; and films. *Hybrid media* are a convergence between the traditional media, digitization, and the internet (Silverblatt 2014: 46). Good examples are the presentation of a film on a flat screen television set, iPads, and smart phones; a film producer who releases a teaser for a new film online; or the uploading of amateur video shots on a cell phone on sites like YouTube (Silverblatt 2014: 46-47). *Digital media* or new media are those that are related to the Internet with digitization comprised of texts, images, graphics, sound, and motion. These digital media are different from the traditional mass media because of their nonlinear interactive features that allow the user to control the pace of the presentation and discover more links to other webpages (Silverblatt et al. 2014: 47). Digital media fall into the category of the mass media as well when the media are roughly categorized into the mass media and personal media. Mass media send a message from one to many receivers. Personal media aids interpersonal communication or group communication.

New media technologies in this contemporary globalization period manifest the age of a mediated society. New media, digital media or online media, consist of media that are based on global internet connections or the World Wide Web (WWW). They include social networking sites such as Facebook, LinkedIn, and VKontakte; video-sharing platforms such as YouTube and XVideos; wikis such as Wikipedia; blogs such as Blogspot, Wordpress, and Blogger; microblogs such as Twitter and Sina Weibo; online pinboards such as Tumblr and Pinterest; and photo-sharing sites such as Instagram (Fuchs & Sandoval 2015: 165). Top ten popular Social Media Sites, as of January 2016, are Facebook, Twitter, LinkedIn, Pinterest, Google Plus+, Tumblr, Instagram, VK, Flickr, and Vine (ebizmba.com 2016). These platforms allow users to create and share texts, images, and motion images among friends and self-defined networks of contacts; they can as well collaboratively create and edit content (Fuchs & Sandoval 2015: 165-166). This is a converging of interpersonal and mass communication. Interpersonal communication has been known to be interactive by one to one communication with feedback loops. Mass communication, using mass media such as radio, television, newspapers, magazines, and Public Service Announcements (PSA), was known as an uni-directional communication, as a message sent from a sender to multiple receivers through book, newspaper, film, radio, or television. The mass media genre can be divided into mainstream media and alternative media. The *mainstream media* are those that operate under commercial control for profit, while alternative media aim at reporting political and social issues to empower citizens and local public sphere to engage in social interactions (Pajnik 2015: 118). *Alternative media* tend to challenge the mainstream media and stand for the rights of the underserved. They are part of the civic society and promote participation and collaboration among like-minded people. Examples of alternative media are indymedia or Independent Media, Wikinews, and Blogs. Indymedia are alternative in that their production processes are based on participation and consensus-sought decision-making. They provide public-access content or open publishing (Hackett 2015: 58-59). Wikinews allows citizen journalists to set their own agenda by publishing their own first-hand reports and offers articles synthesized from other media sources (Hackett 2015: 59). Wikis are a type of websites that allow users to add on already published content just like in Wikipedia (TechTarget 2015). Blogs allow citizen journalists to blossom. Heinonen and Domingo (2008: 7-11) explain four types of blogs: citizen blogs, audience blogs, journalist blogs, and media blogs. Citizen blogs are written by people from outside the media organization. In other words, amateurs, or so-called citizen journalists, write them. Audience blogs are what the media institutions allow the public to write under the condition that the organizations can moderate and facilitate the blogs. Journalist blogs are blogs written by journalists outside the rubric of media institutions. Media blogs are written by journalists working in media institutions.

Mass-Self Communication

In this mediated society, we are now part of a digital network. We are the mass media--when we receive a message and send it out to many people in a network. We also function as interpersonal communicators both offline and online, in real time and chosen time. Elias (1978: 15) introduces the term, "communicative figuration," to describe individuals' networks which constitute the process of interweaving actions among the socials at a different scale such as a family, a group, the state or society. Hepp (2013: 93) uses Elias' term to describe the social reciprocal interaction in the digital era. Hepp (2013: 94) explains that a figuration can be scattered on many local spaces – *translocal* is the term he uses. For instance, at the family level the communicative figuration consists of smart or cell phones, digital photo albums, letters, postcards, and watching TV together. National or transnational communicative figurations are called public spheres and are comprised of traditional mass media, WikiLeaks, Twitter and blogs, and the media of the social web (Hepp 2013: 94). These examples explain how interpersonal communication, mass communication, and individuals function as a mass medium in an interweaving fashion. Castells (2013:55) calls the process an individual operates within the communicative figuration "mass self-communication." Castells (2013:55) also describes the way one can reach a global audience by posting a video on YouTube, a blog with RSS links to a number of web sources, or a message to a massive e-mail list. At the same time, one can perform self-communication by self-generating messages and self-directing the messages to potential receivers, and self-selecting or self-retrieving messages or content from the World Wide Web and electronic communication.

MEDIATIZATION

Communicative figurations have helped create a virtual community and virtual experiences, at the same time they have been a woven thread of the globalization process, therefore, created a global consciousness, by which people compare their own living conditions with that of others (McQuail 2005: 51-52). Thompson (1995: 174) goes further and argues that people can appropriate global cultural products to their local situation. The term, hybridity or hybrid media culture, emerged as a result of the global-local interaction or glocalization process.

New media usage in many countries has raised concerns about threats to national values, privacy, security, laws, and influences from major soft power producers in the world. The process whereby culture and society are increasingly dependent on the media and their logic, in such a way that the degree of the social interactions within a given culture and society is modulated by media capital, is called *mediatization* (Hjarvard 2013:17). Mediatization is seen as a longer term process than mediation, as the media's influence on the change of the social and institutional interactions is to be expected, whereas the mediation describes only the concrete act of communication by using a type of media in a given social context (Hjarvard 2013: 18-19).

Mediatization can have impacts on culture by increasing general information about the citizens of the world and cultures; accelerating contact with peoples who possess "the otherness"; enhancing contact with people within the same culture for support; redefining one's own identity and think of identity management; and widening the gap of access to communication technology, or the so-called digital divide (Martin and Nakayama 2004: 6). These aspects together with the changing of immigration patterns and demographics result in culturally diverse societies across the globe.

MEDIA LITERACY

Traditional mass media was known as the spin-doctoring industry, as they have created hypes on agendas, celebrities, and political issues. By doing so the mass media have power to influence the rise and fall of political leaders, disseminate, promote, or suppress, information or ideas (Louw 2005: 26). Louw (2005: 59-92) explains further that, as a result of commercial pressures, the mediatization process has affected the construction of reality by gatekeeping information and agenda setting in such a way that the audiences are being manipulated by the journalists' values and ideology. Thus, objectivity does not exist. That is reiterated by the fact that the mass media operate within a certain political and commercial environment.

As we have seen in *Chapter 2,* communication is the process we construct and share meanings via social interaction. The media are not the message, but the genre and format of the media characterize the message. For instance, news in a newspaper can be more in-depth than on television. News on websites is shorter than news in a newspaper to prevent the reader from scrolling down too much. Hence, there is less investigative online news available. However, this can be compensated with video clips or audio files of interviews on demand.

With the emerging of new media, optimistic views about the possibilities of power distribution, interactive two-way communication, and democratization are being discussed. In 2005, Louw (2005: 124) presented his skeptical view about the new media arguing that the audience still trusted the traditional mass media as their sources of information.

In 2013, however, Castells reports the power of the multi-media network or media convergence on changes in organization and culture. According to Share (2015: 211-212), media convergence can be seen at three levels. The first level is about a hardware device that can have multiple functions, such as a smart phone that can take and send images and videos, play music, send and receive text messages, download and upload content online, play games, and chat. The second level is about the media conglomerate that combines many media companies so that the media owner can control more different types of services and contents. The third level is about a synergy between two or more different industries. The joint-ventures may consist of a combination of knowledge and information, consumerism, popular culture, entertainment, and education. A good example is a synergy of news, politics, and entertainment.

It is a must that health communicators be media-literate. Media literacy, according to Turow's definition, is "the ability to access, analyze, evaluate and communicate messages in a variety of forms" (Turow 2014: 20-21). To develop media literacy skills, one must understand the following concepts:

- *What we see in the media is constructed reality.* Media are not like transparent windows through which we can look at the world without bias. During media production, media messages and images are created, shaped, and positioned and that involves many decisions as to what should be selected and presented to serve a specific purpose. Even though they look like a natural reflection of reality, media are influenced by business decisions and constraints.
- *The mass media are produced and influenced by commercial organization.* Therefore, media have commercial implications. Media are organized to gain profits and power. A large media company is more likely than a small one to take advantage of media convergence. That means the large company has more power to control the media production, distribution, and exhibition. This is undemocratic and threatens the independence and diversity of information, and that creates the possibility to dominate another culture with so-called "soft power."
- *The media operate within a political environment.* We should be aware that this environment deeply influences the media content on ideology, point of views, and values.

- *The format of the media*, e.g., the television, the movie, the magazine, the blog, the VDO clip etc., shapes its presentation, content, characteristics, codes, and convention.
- *Audiences negotiate meaning in media*. Different audiences interpret the same media message differently. They show that they are active recipients of the media by letting the communicators know via many feedback channels.
- *Each medium has a unique aesthetic form*.
- *The media reflect the society's visions*.
  (Turow 2014: 21-22, Share 2015: 23-32).

Media literacy can be taught at school and be integrated throughout the curriculum. It can be categorized into visual literacy, aural literacy, multimedia literacy, and alternative media literacy (Share 2015: 192-197). For visual literacy, it is to understand that different lighting, camera angles, lenses, colors, distance between object and the cameras, types of camera, and object composition create a different story. For aural literacy, it is to understand that the same sentence connotes a different meaning depending on the context in which they are spoken and heard (Share 2015: 194). Music as sound effects can add meaningful interpretation to the media content (Share 2015: 194). Multimedia literacy, knowing how to form ideas, create a storyboard for digital storytelling, writing script, drawing illustrations, preparing images and video clips, recording sounds, and assembling all the elements in a PowerPoint or a short film is a good exercise of participatory production that a group of people can take part in (Share 2015:195-196). Alternative media literacy is how to analyze the hegemony of the mainstream media on gender, race, class, sexuality, etc. and produce or look at the world from underprivileged perspectives. Or see how power from a dominant ideology is represented in mainstream media content (Share 2015: 197).

As summarized from Share (2015: 195-196), it is important to learn to differentiate scientific fact from fiction in popular culture. It is helpful to learn how graphs and infographics can distort information. For social media, it is also important to differentiate hoax websites from informative ones. It is a challenge to implant social justice in media education. This implies that media ethics is part of media literacy.

US corporations are now using green marketing as a public relations strategy to sell sustainability. We should be aware that, sometimes, green product advertising deflects the claim that its product is ecologically friendly. Consumers have to be aware of the loose standard of green labels that can be deceptive, such as free range or cage free eggs, report Cox and Pezzullo (2016: 268-269). Cox and Pezzullo (2016: 270) also report on green image enhancements; for instance "the use of PR (public relations) to improve the brand or ethos of the corporation itself by associating it with positive environmental messages, practices, and products." They also explain that corporate image repairs are like crisis management to restore a company's reputation that was tarnished by any wrong doing to the environment (Cox & Pezzullo 2016: 274-275).

The more advanced the Web-based technologies are, the more we are confronted with privacy issues. Critics may argue that some discreet information and private records may be exposed to online marketers or advertisement companies and, in the worst case, to hackers and abusers. Also the use of social media can tarnish the image or even the career for those who love self-expression beyond the limit. Cyber bullying, 'lurking' and the spreading of false information is on the rise. Collecting information of a personal nature should only be done when that person is properly informed. Then the collector would allow the audience to have informed consent and gives them the opportunity to refuse (Turner 2014: 188).

Community Media for Health Communication

Community media emerged as an alternative to the limitations of the mainstream media, particularly television, with the core idea that communication works best within a local context and when it is created by locals for locals (Prasad 2009 a: 222). Community media consist of electronic media with feedback loops; new media which allows interactivities or a combination of electronic media and new media; folk media such as theatre play, traditional storytelling performances, music and dance; print media such as posters, banners, pamphlets, brochures; and of course personal media--health communicators. Popular media used in community empowerment are community radio which allows talkback phone-ins, community television which allows the public to create content and receives feedbacks via its multi-media website, community-based on-line telematics systems, community videos, digital storytelling, and social media networks.

In order to let the grassroots participate in healthcare reform or community health and wellness or disease prevention, community media are known to be used in *Participatory Action Research (PAR)* which is a process that integrates community health development, development journalism, and indigenous knowledge communication systems (Manyozo 2012: 247). PAR is a process which requires inputs and collaboration from the stakeholders and researcher/health communicator to design research, collect data, analyze data, and evaluation of the whole process in order to improve on each step for better outcomes (will be explained in detail in *Chapter 7*).

Community media are tools that health communicators, who act as health advocates or health mobilizers, use to engage local intellects, stakeholders, and community leaders to the transformation of community polity to be a driving force to facilitate health and development initiatives (Manyozo 2012: 247). Community health development is related to power from the grassroots; development journalism is related to power as collective decision making; and indigenous knowledge communication systems are related to power as the articulation of the local wisdom and oral skills (Manyozo 2012: 247). Media advocacy in health issues is the strategic use of the mass and mass-self media to raise issues and mobilize participation and actions aiming at public health policy and structural change to advance and maintain health and well-being in communities.

Community media can be used to alert, amplify, and engage the stakeholders in advocacy campaigns or social mobilizing campaigns to increase awareness and urge action on environmental problems that can indirectly affect our health. One of the problems we are facing is the relationship between fossil fuels and climate change. In a combined fashion, global warming has been caused by a buildup of gases, carbon dioxide emitted from fossil fuel combustion and other gases known as greenhouse gases, which traps warmth from the sun (Goldberg 2014: 55). The topics of campaigns can range from clean power, sustainability infrastructure, zero waste, renewable energy, climate justice, mercury poisoning in fish, etc. (Goldberg 2014).

As it is known that health-related problems are the consequence of power inequalities, media advocacy does not only concern with media actions to put pressure on decision-makers, but it also helps build up the power and the formation of coalitions and grassroots actions necessary for lobbying (Prasad 2009 a: 85). Advocacy can be managed by information activities: traditionally, such as lobbying with decision makers through personal contacts and direct mails; holding seminars, rallies and newsmaking events; ensuring regular newspaper, magazine, television, and radio coverage and getting endorsement from celebrities or key people in international agencies (Prasad 2009 a: 86). New media advocacy is done by using social media such as Twitter, Facebook, Instagram, e-mails, websites, and online text messaging. Participatory-based media advocacy is what we are aiming for in a community to have the locals participating in the management and content production. Health communication for structural and social change can be achieved by ways of using a multi-media strategy which combines old and new media of which the production are participatory-based started at a community scale first.

Detailed information on each community medium will be discussed next.

Community Radio

Community radio refers to a low power radio station. Radio is suitable for developing countries to communicate about health and diseases, because it is inexpensive to run or to get a receiver. Furthermore, it bypasses the literacy barrier. Community radio can start up initiative to have the audience participate in program production and it can be used to empower local audiences to be health active. A feedback mechanism by phone-ins or talk-backs or even letters from the listeners is encouraged to have for two-way communication. As well, participatory social marketing by using radio drama or storytelling, in the form of edutainment, can be used to turn the community awareness on health policy, health practices, disease prevention, environmental problems such as climate change and more, including food safety and nutrition, growing organic food for consumption, health literacy, etc. A survey or rating analysis of programs can be conducted to get feedbacks.

Community Television

Same as community radio, community television is a powerful communication tool to bypass the literacy barrier. Community television is a good source to offer program production by way of participation of the stakeholders on healthcare policy, or health and/or environmental information and problem discussion. It is a good channel for public minorities to participate and have their voice heard. Participatory social marketing on television, in the form of edutainment on health and diseases, can be produced to empower the community on a specific topic. As well, it can be used to air forums of discussion on the same topics as radio but it can broadcast a (on consensus) selection of films and documentary films related to disease prevention, health issues and social problems, exercise, organic farming, sustainable agriculture, etc. to educate and empower the community dwellers. It can also broadcast folk songs, music, and dance, and theatre plays to empower the community on the issues of environmental health and public health.

Participants in community television should be trained on basic TV production provided by the station in order to being able to handle TV cameras, edit with editing programs such as FinalCutPro, manipulate and create images with Photoshop, and to conduct interviews. The station should have a multimedia website to upload broadcast programs for the audience to download and watch on demand and to provide feedback. Surveys and regular interviews of the audience on the quality of programs should be conducted.

Community Video

Community video is cheaper than community television. Developing countries have long made use of this tool. Videos can be recorded with a hand-held video camera or mobile phone. Using an editing program to compile a video according to a storyboard can be participatory work among a group of interested stakeholders with the facilitation of health communicators. Video clips can be played on a laptop or video projectors to empower people on health and environment or mobilize them for a change in policy. Feedbacks can be gained by interaction between the audience and the video presenter/health communicator, interviews, telephones, or a survey.

Community-Based Telematics Systems

These can be telematics warning systems on environmental disasters, such as Tsunami warning systems or telematics warning on pollution levels in the air.

Community Tradition/Folklore Media

The folk media are spontaneous expressions of culture; they invite dialogues between the performers and the audience (Prasad 2009 a: 190). They can be strategically combined with mass media to raise awareness on health.

Folk media include puppetry, songs, theatre plays, performances, folk singers, and music bands to help convey health promotion messages or disease awareness or to discuss dilemmas regarding HIV/AIDS. They can be used to promote health practices, hygiene, and knowledge on diseases. Video clips of performances can be uploaded on the community website and/or broadcast via community television. Or it can be recorded as video clips and played on a projector for community discussion.

Street theatre units in India staged performances around women's rights, dowry, domestic violence, child abuse, and literacy (Prasad 2009 a: 191). In Thailand they are used to voice the rights of HIV living people, children's rights, democracy and so forth.

Community Print Media

These include billboards, banners, posters, newsletters, local newspapers, pamphlets, wall news, etc. The objective is to provide information to the locals. Participatory production is the essence of being a community print media. Writing, editing skills, and desktop publishing skills can be trained so that the locals can present the health and environmental issues from their own perspective. Newsletter and newspaper have been proven effective in India and elsewhere (Prasad 2009 a: 164-166). Feedback can be given by letters to the editor, phone calls, e-mails, and online replies.

Community Alternative Media

Alternative media can be mobile exhibitions, broadcast towers in a rural village, signs on taxis and busses, sandwich men, public health volunteers, opinion leaders in the community, and religious leaders. As adapted from Kakar (1987: 131-132) in Prasad (2009 a: 448), communication channels to be used in communication campaigns could be:

- Places of mass exposure--such as bus stops, railway platforms, etc.
- Temporary gatherings—weekly bazaars, fairs and meals, religious gatherings.
- Mobile bus panels, rail panels, horse carts, taxies, cycle rickshaws, bullock carts, special rail exhibitions.
- Educational material—money orders, post cards, envelopes, transport tickets, aerogrammes.
- Audio media—mp3 players, podcasts, audiovisual vans.
- Mass media—radio, press (newspapers/magazines), touring cinemas, cinema theatres, rural/agricultural press, outdoor sites.
- High technology media—satellite TV, TV ground stations, cable TV.
- Interpersonal media—auxiliary nurses, midwives, family planning workers, village leaders, schoolteachers, postmasters.

Community New Media

In the contemporary globalization, digital media or new media can help the underserved to voice their concerns and the general public to access health information for decision making on health and wellness, diseases, and well-being. New media differ from traditional media in a way that they offer interactivities. Information and Communications Technologies or ICT are synergies of information technology and telecommunications, which include hardware, software, and networks. Verma (2011: 4) explains "ICT consists of IT as well as telephony, broadcast media, and all types of audio and video processing and transmission." ICT has been used in medicine, health care, sustainable development, climate change, biodiversity, and other areas.

E-health, Web 2.0, Web 3.0, and Web 4.0 are the topics of debate and discussion in the area of ICT for healthcare. Before the emergence of e-health in 2000, telemedicine as a delivery of healthcare from a distance via telecommunication technology was used (Kivits 2013: 215). For sustainability, the use of telemedicine for preventive efforts and patient education is still relevant even though e-health is becoming more and more popular.

Telemedicine is the use of telecommunications technologies for a distance prognosis, medical coaching and consultation for the benefits of patients who live far away from the medical resources and facilities (Turner 2003: 516). That can be contacts among medical specialists only or between a medical specialist and a patient. Turner (2003: 517-518) explains that telemedicine technologies are comprised of telephone, fax machine, interactive video conferencing, e-mail, and Web-based interactions. They are used for specific diseases such as tumors, fractures, lesions, heart murmur, etc. Specialty areas are in psychiatry, dermatology, cardiology, general surgery, etc. and that created new terms such as telepsychiatry, teleoncology, telepathololgy, and teledermatology. Telemedicine can be used to help with clinical problem solving such as routine consultation and second opinion, transmission of diagnostic images and other medical data, preventive medicine, public health and patient education, etc. In India, telemedicine facilities rely on low bandwidth technology in remote areas to cut down on a patient's travel to doctor for a referral or reports.

According to Kivits (2013: 213-224), E-health has connected all medical parties: health professionals, institutions, patients, and the general public in an interactive fashion; and that has improved cure possibilities. Next, E-health in the form of virtual health has brought all health-concerned public together to form a virtual community to voice their concerns. Further, websites on health and medicine have mushroomed over the past decade. Information on health is now readily available to the public. However, health information seekers are not necessarily patients, and not all available online health information is accurate or trustworthy.

Internet radio, Web radio or e-radio is a broadcasting service (or Netcasting) that makes use of the Internet connection and has been increasingly controlled by media conglomerates (Prasad 2009: 234-235). It is a convergence of the Internet and broadcasting which can be used to display photos or graphics, text and links, and real-time or received-time feedback channels, such as chat rooms and message boards (Prasad 2009 a: 234-235). This tool enhances the access of information and interactions for/about health and environment impact on health in a community.

Internet television or Internet TV or e-TV is a convergence of television and the Internet. It can be watched on a regular TV set (via a set-top box), or on a computer, or on a portable device such as a mobile phone. It allows the viewer to have Video-on-Demand (Prasad 2009 a: 237). It is an interactive or passive medium. It can be used to transmit local development and health issues.

Geographic Information System (GIS) is a collection of computer hardware, software, and geographical data for a community database system. GIS data can be used under the health and environment implications such as for tracking illegal dumpsites, monitoring abuses against the elderly, women, and children.

Prasad (2009 a: 175) reports that in a rural community in India, a community information center (CIC) or telecenter is part of an initiative to bridge the digital divide. The government or an NGO helps set up an ICT point together with a copying machine, telephone booths, and a computer with software. The midwives can help entering demographic data and help with family planning. Such wired villages in India have become habitable ones with medical facilities.

The prospect of participation within the virtual community is brighter since the introduction of the Web 2.0 by DiNucci in 1999 and this concept was popularized by O'Reilly and Dougherty at the O'Reilly MediaWeb 2.0 Conference in late 2004 (O'ReillyMedia Inc. 2015). It is the second stage development of the World Wide Web. It is different from the traditional World Wide Web in the sense that it allows inputs from the users on the Web content, thus, increases more collaborative interactivity than the Web1.0 which allowed users to only browse and read the content (TechTarget 2015). It can be called a dynamic Web instead of the traditional static World Wide Web. TechTarget website lists the following elements of Web 2.0:

1) Wikis: websites that allow users to add on and edit site content.
2) Software such as a Service (SaaS), webapps, and cloud computing: applications that service providers or software venders provide to the customers through a browser interface on the internet.
3) Nomadicity: access to Wi-Fi networks with the mobile computing function that allows smartphones, tablets, and other mobile devices to connect to readily accessible Wi-Fi networks.
4) Mash-ups: web pages or applications that extract elements from two or more sources and integrate them.
5) Social networking sites: Facebook, Twitter, LinkedIn, and Google+
6) Crowdsourcing, crowdfunding, and crowdsource testing: the ability to outsource tasks, project funding or investment, beta-type software to a large number of external people for the purpose of helping executing tasks, donation or co-invest, or testing software with a large group of participants.
7) User-generated content (UGC): allows the users to write, post image, sound, and motion files online.
8) Unified communications (UC): allows the users to integrate multiple forms of call and multi-media and cross media messages.
9) Social curation: allows the users to share content organized around one or more themes or topics. Examples of social curation sites are Instagram, Reddit, Pinterest, and Digg.

In the near future, we are expecting the further development of Web 3.0 and Web 4.0. Web 3.0 is another step of development of Web 2.0. According to About.com (2015 b), it was coined by Markoff of the New York Times in 2006. Web 3.0 offers semantic web which all information can be categorized, stored, and understood by both human and computer. A combination of semantic web and artificial intelligence is expected. The other distinctive feature of Web 3.0 is the availability of virtual reality worlds. It offers the merging of entertainment systems and mobile internet devices. Internet access on mobile devices (cell phones, smartphones, pocket PCs) will be as popular as text messaging. Web 3.0 opens the doors to connecting more data, be it big data, open data, or personal data. Web 4.0, also known as WebOS, refers to the super intelligent web that allows flowing of data from one platform to another with only one single operating system. More merging of and personalized data will be expected (Paul-Edwards 2013). As summarized from PCWorld.com (2015), with the upcoming Web 4.0 in the future, the moving to intelligent robots which can be commanded by human thought is possible. This leads to medically focused devices such as the retina implant chip and Cyberkinetics. Radio frequency identification tags which allow interactions between humans and machines will be controlled by Web 4.0, and in the near future machines can send data to one another and let us know the results.

WHAT ARE THE IMPLICATIONS FOR ALL OF THESE ADVANCED NEW MEDIA TECHNOLOGIES FOR HEALTH COMMUNICATION?

By now, it is clear that E-health has progressed from didactic patient information websites and telemedicine to "participant-centered approaches including websites, blogs, wikis, mobile phones, e-mail, video, and podcasts, and electronic medical records" (Suggs & Ratzan 2012: 251). Not only do participants search for health information online, they have become health agents who share and promote an individual expression of health experience by using the interconnected e-health networks. However, it is advisable to keep in mind that individuals experience health and illnesses differently due to their specific context and other economic-sociocultural factors, such as income or living conditions.

Health literacy promoted by e-health helps informed patients, health-competent consumers, and the general public to make optimal economic health decisions, to save money from unnecessary healthcare expenses (Suggs & Ratzon 2012: 256). The first step of health literacy is helping individuals so that they are better informed about treatment outcomes; more likely to adopt and adhere to preventive regimes; recognize warning signs of serious diseases and seek necessary healthcare services; follow instructions from healthcare providers better; know how to use medicines correctly; are not afraid to ask questions regarding health and healthcare and by doing so help reduce medical error risks and increase adherence to provider's advice (Suggs & Ratzan 2012: 257).

The development of Web 2.0 and beyond aids participation possibilities for stakeholders to start up a virtual community or a physical community so that every stakeholder gets connected. Suggs and Ratzan (2012: 258) report about social media in health. There are, for instance, PatientsLikeMe, which is a social networking platform for patients all over the world; the FAN project (Family, Activity, and Nutrition), funded by the local Public Health Department, and Health Promotion Switzerland to connect parents and young children with social media platform using Wordpress to share texts, images, videos, e-mails, SMS reinforcement to improve their diet and exercises; FanSpace in Australia is about sexual health and safer sex to young people and men who have sex with men; and so forth. *Mobile Health* or m-health is another version of e-health via mobile technologies. That allows access to people with tailored messages and complementing messages by print, radio, television, and the Internet in order to facilitate consultations of patients with healthcare providers; provide text messages on health information, prevention, and care; disease surveillance; and disease monitoring (Suggs & Ratzan 2012: 259). Mobile phones with SMS (text communication with a maximum of 160 characters) or MMS (images, videos, audio, and rich text) facilities can be used to promote awareness of health-risk behaviors (Suggs & Ratzan 2012: 260).

For health mobilizers or health advocates, it is interesting to make use of virtual health communities via social media in combination with mobile phones to voice for an improvement of health policies or other health-related concerns of the general public to the policy makers. Global health policy has shifted from government funded to more private health systems. That may counter some national priorities, where health is valued as a public good rather than as a commodity for those who can afford it (Verma 2011: 52). If human rights include the right to have access to proper healthcare for underserved communities, healthcare equality advocacy would be one on the top of agendas for sustainable development. A change of health policy will be the best lasting impact e-health can make in the contemporary globalization period.

Health mobilizers or health advocates can as well make use of e-health together with m-health to boost up health literacy among the stakeholders to make them realize that information seeking about health online is only a primary step. Health assessments or examinations by a physician should be performed every five years for adults over 18 until age 40, and every one to three years thereafter; those who take prescription medications need more frequent assessments (Emedicinehealth.com 2015 b). Credibility of websites about health and medicine should be one of the crossing areas of health and communication literacy that health communicators must know about.

Having a community website which everyone in a community can interact with, and voice their concerns and suggestions, should be a good way towards a participatory democracy and to mobilize for social justice in healthcare. Topics for discussion are similar to those already mentioned for radio and television. The website of a community can be best multimedia and allow open access for content collaboration from community dwellers. If the level of media literacy of a community is not good enough, the website should embed an interactive program for the inhabitants to learn online. Any information on health or digital storytelling, or video clips produced by the locals can be selected and uploaded on the website. Any feedback channel should as well embed such as blogs, Q&A, questions to the administrator of the website, etc. Feedbacks can be voice messages, or print messages, in addition to online messages.

Blogging can be another channel that health communicators engage in with online communities. An interesting and inexpensive medium are Podcasts (only audio) or Vodcasts (both audio and video). Podcast/Vodcast production concerns production of video and/or audio files that are episodic, downloadable, and program driven in order to be fed automatically with computer software (Barker et al. 2013: 105). Podcasts can be directly played off the website on a computer, downloaded to a computer and listened to offline, and downloaded to portable MP3 players for listening offline. Participatory podcast or vodcast production is possible.

Another tool for engaging discussion on health is a Webinar or teleseminar (Barker et al. 2013: 114). It is a web-based seminar which is interactive in nature. To attend a webinar, the listener can call a phone number or listen live through the internet. Live-stream video and slide presentations can be presented during webinars. This technology is promising as a participatory-based medium.

Conclusion

Old and new media can be strategically integrated to advocate health literacy, health and well-being, health and a clean environment, and social justice and equality in healthcare. Community media could be seen as tools to alert and amplify health and environmental issues that affect health and engage the locals for actions and health behaviors. The media alone cannot change the culture and mobilize the locals. Health communicators should be media literate in order to facilitate the interactions about/for health in a meaningful way. Health communicators should be good facilitators in participatory-based media production content as well.

Communication strategies will be discussed in the next chapter.

REFERENCES

Castells, M. (2013). *Communication Power*. Oxford, U.K: Oxford University Press.

Cox, R. & Pezzullo, P. (2016). *Environmental Communication and the Public Sphere* (4th ed.) Los Angelis-London-New Dehli-Singapore-Washington DC-Boston: Sage.

Paul-Edwards, J. (2013). What might Web 4.0 Look Like and Should You be Preparing? IMedia Connection website (http://www.imediaconnection.com/content/34206.asp, accessed on November 2nd, 2015).

Elias, N. (1978). *What is Sociology?* London: Hutchinson.

Fuchs, C. & Sandoval, M. (2015). The Political Economy of Capitalist and Alternative Social Media. In C. Atton (Ed.) *The Routledge Companion to Alternative and Community Media*. London-New York: Routledge.

Goldberg, R. (2014). *Understanding Contemporary Social Problems through Media*. Boulder-London: Paradigm Publishers.

Hackett, R. A. & Gurleyen, P. (2015). Beyond the Binaries? Alternative Media and Objective Journalism. In C. Atton (Ed.) *The Routledge Companion to Alternative and Community Media*. London-New York: Routledge.

Heinonen, A. & Domingo, D. (2008). Webblogs and Journalism: A Typology to Explore the Blurring Boundaries. *Nordicom Review*, 29(1), 3-15.

Hepp, A. (2013). *Cultures of Mediatization*. (K. Tribe Trans.) Cambridge: Polity Press.

Hjarvard, S. (2013). *The Mediatization of Culture and Society*. Routledge: London and New York.

Kakar, V. N. (1987). *Communication in India's Family Planning—India's Experience*. New Delhi: National Institute of Health and Family Welfare.

Kivits, J. (2013). E-health and Renewed Sociological Approaches to Health and Illness. In K. Orton-Johnson & N. Prior (Eds.) *Digital Sociology. Critical Perspectives*. New York: Palgrave Macmillan., pp.213-226.

Louw, E. (2005). *The Media and Political Process*. London-Thousand Oaks-New Dehli: Sage Publications.

Manyozo, L. (2012). Community Media, Health Communication, and Engagement. A Theoretical Matrix. In R. Obregon & S. Waisbord (Eds.) *The Handbook of Global Health Communication*. West Sussex: Wiley-Blackwell, pp. 233-250.

Martin, J. N. & Nakayama, T. K. (2004). *Intercultural Communication in Contexts*. McGraw Hill: Boston.

McQuail, D. (2005). *McQuail's Mass Communication Theory*. (5th ed.). London-Thousand Oaks-New Delhi: Sage Publications.

Pajnik, M. (2015). Changing Citizenship, Practising (Alternative) Politics. In C. Atton (Ed.) *The Routledge Companion to Alternative and Community Media*. London and New York: Routledge, pp. 113-122.

Prasad, K. (2009 a). *Communication for Development. Reinventing Theory and Action. Volume 1. Understanding Communication*. Delhi: B.R. Publishing Corporation.

Share, J. (2015). *Media Literacy is Elementary. Teaching Youth to Critically Read and Create Media* (2nd ed.). New York: Peter Lang.

Silverblatt, A., Smith, A., Miller, D., Smith, J. et al. (2014). *Media Literacy. Keys to Interpreting Media Messages* (4th ed.). Santa Barbara, CA: Praeger.

Suggs, L. S. & Ratzan, S. C. (2012). Global E-health Communication. In R. Obregon & S. Waisbord (Eds.) *The Handbook of Global Health Communication*. West Sussex: Wiley-Blackwell, pp. 251-273.

Turner, J. W. (2003). Telemedicine: Expanding Health Care into Virtual Environments. In T. L. Thompson, A. Dorsey, K. I. Miller & R. Parrott (Eds.) *Handbook of Health Communication*. New York-London: Lawrence Erlbaum Associates, pp. 515-535.

Thompson, J. (1995). *The Media and Modernity. A Social Theory of the Media*. Cambridge: Polity Press.

Turow, J. (2014). *Media Today (5th ed.)*. New York-London: Routledge.

Verma, S. (2011). *International Media Communication in a Global Age*. Jaipur: Prateeksha Publications.

Websites

About.com 2015 b
http://webtrends.about.com/od/web20/a/what-is-web-30.htm, accessed on November 2nd, 2015.

Ebizmba.com 2016
http://www.ebizmba.com/articles/social-networking-websites, accessed on January 20th, 2016.

Emedicinehealth.com 2015 b
http://www.emedicinehealth.com/checkup/article_em.htm#a_checkup_how_often, accessed on November 1st, 2015.

IMedia Connection 2015
http://www.imediaconnection.com/content/34206.asp, accessed on November 2nd, 2015.

TechTarget (2015)
http://whatis.techtarget.com/definition/crowdsource-testing, accessed on November 2nd, 2015.

O'Reilly Media Inc. 2015
http://www.oreilly.com/pub/a/web2/archive/what-is-web-20.html, accessed on November 2nd, 2015.

PCWorld 2015
http://www.pcworld.com/article/143110/article.html, accessed on November 2nd, 2015.

Chapter 7

HEALTH COMMUNICATION STRATEGIES FOR SUSTAINABILITY: THE PRINCIPLES

ABSTRACT

This chapter integrates the previous chapters regarding relevant theories under the multiplicity paradigm, external and internal factors that have impacts on health and diseases, media literacy and knowledge on the mass media, and new media and community media to devise appropriate communication strategies by deploying the Participatory Action Research (PAR) method. The major component of the strategies emphasized in this chapter will be participatory-based communication. The aims are to advocate or mobilize "health" to change the environment and to accommodate health behavior, rather than using messages only to persuade or demand health behavioral change of individuals without thinking about a healthy environment. This has proven to be a sustainable way to health for all.

Keywords: participatory action research, health communication strategies, health communication approaches, types of health issues, communication as part of a social media network

INTRODUCTION

It is clear by now that health communication underpinned by the multiplicity paradigm emphasizes the importance of an enabling environment, supported by many theories to encourage individuals to change their health behaviors, as well as health messages and communication. Health messages would not trigger deep down to the behavioral level if they were sent by mass media or new media only, unless they were, as well, amplified and/or modified by group communication or organizational communication. No matter how advanced communications technologies may be, they can only ease access to information and ensure the coverage of messages; they cannot replace the 'human touch' or the importance of actors/personal media to win over the heart of the stakeholders.

In a world of information overload, people go through a mass of messages every day. They filter relevant messages through their black box/internal gatekeeping/cognitive system.

The messages they retain, according to social psychologists, would be the ones that reinforce their own beliefs and predispositions (see *Chapter 2*). However, that sort of information will trigger the awareness of the stakeholder, alter their attitude or eventually change their health behavior when audiences gained some advice or had discussed it with other people, and they would change their behavior when they see fit. That means when knowledge or awareness matches someone's personal needs, amplified by environmental factors, that person will reach what health communicators call "*self-efficacy*" or the ability to change one's health behavior. Health behaviors will be maintained when the infrastructure supports them. As many services or facilities cannot be offered by civic groups, they must be provided by the state authority, such as a local healthcare service station, a nearby marketplace that offers a variety of fresh foods and fruits, a recreation area, or a good health education curriculum at school. As well, the state should take care of the supra-structural change, meaning enacting laws to ensure clean air to breath, clean water to consume, food safety, traffic rule enforcement, and so on. All of these cannot be achieved without civil advocacy, preferably, a participatory-based advocacy or mobilization for social action. In other words, voicing the concerns and suggestions from the grassroots level up to the policymakers. Communication arts and skills are indispensable to aid with the advocacy or social mobilization process.

To make communication for/about health a success, we need a strategy: a plan of action that would ensure the long-term goals. Strategic planning involves specific stages of defining the health problem/need; setting goals and objectives that can be assessed during a short- or long-term; identifying resources, including financial and human ones; preparing a plan of action, including media selection and social networking; budgeting; and setting up 'monitoring and evaluation' (M&E) mechanisms (Karl 1999: 100).

A health communication strategy for sustainability aims at health equity or social justice in health, while respecting human rights and ethics as long-term goals. Short-term measurable goals must be identified, as well as medium and long-term goals that require qualitative assessments. Next, they will also need to plan to scope down a program or a project to a number of related mini/sub-projects to guarantee the workability of those projects (Karl 1999: 101). This means that the applicability of a project is very important. Aspiration must be compromised with limited budgets, human resources, and media available, including other external factors and unexpected circumstances. Strategic planning for health advocacy needs to identify partners for collaborative action; targets of change, either people or institutions; arguments and counter arguments in advance (Karl 1999: 101). Sending many messages through multiple media channels during a cross-sectional time frame only will not make a health communication campaign a sustainable one. Health communicators as health mobilizers or health advocates need to pay attention to both online and off-line campaigns. That requires participation and group effort of all stakeholders concerned. Health communicators should consider methodologies to gather and evaluate data, and to analyze media contents. Indicators for sustainability for health, education, governance, and environment: actors, levels of analysis and implementation, different development communication approaches, channels, processes, methods, and messages need to be taken into account as explained in *chapter 5*.

Let's now explain these theoretical concepts by way of practical health communication strategies.

HEALTH COMMUNICATION STRATEGIES FOR SUSTAINABLE DEVELOPMENT

To attain health at all stages of life is a fundamental right for everyone. Sustainability in health is one of the keystones of sustainable development, as good health is an asset and a source of economic and social stability (Chan 2013: 6). Health communication can help accomplish the strategic objectives for sustainability in relation to four interlinked and mutually supportive areas: (a) improving health through a life-course and empowering people; (b) tackling local major health challenges of non-communicable and communicable diseases; (c) strengthening people-centered health systems, public health capacity and emergency preparedness, surveillance and response; and (d) creating resilient communities and supportive environments (WHO Europe 2013: 15). Health communicators can play a facilitating role and address these four priorities while advocating for good governance, health equity, and well-being. Group process or group work and networking is important to enhance critical thinking and creativity, address global health-related problems while strengthening local efforts, and increase people's potential for advocating health equity and mobilizing their health status.

Participatory Action Research (PAR) has been used to improve health and decrease health inequalities through a process in which a researcher and empowered stakeholders together are engaged in identifying and prioritizing problems, planning and implementing the research process, and evaluating improvements and identifying and prioritizing problems. In this ongoing loop, the boundary between the researcher and the researched is quite blurred. It is considered an ongoing and active process that requires a dynamic distribution of power and collaboration in a community. PAR, underpinned by the critical theory and constructivism paradigm, relies on both qualitative and quantitative methods (Baum, MacDougall & Smith 2006: 854). In the very beginning PAR was mainly deployed for evaluating health services in developing countries, but it has been used increasingly in mental health research in developed countries as well (Baum, MacDougall & Smith 2006: 855).

Listed below is a set of logical steps for a health communication strategy, as adapted from Winsemius (1986) by Servaes and Malikhao (2010: 46):

1) Stake holder analysis;
2) Recognizing and defining the public health problem in a community;
3) Setting goals and objectives;
4) Identifying resources; and
5) Maintaining control of the public health problem.

1. STAKEHOLDER ANALYSIS

Using group discussion to examine the interests and roles of various stakeholders including those to whom health related messages are being provided and whose needs are being advocated (Karl 1999: 60-61). A project that engages many local community members would be considered a more sustainable one (Servaes et al. 2012: 24).

2. Recognizing and Defining the Public Health Problem in a Community

This can be done to develop sensitivity and listening skills. Listen to stories told by stakeholders of how they handled problems in the past. Using group discussion to identify problems requires tools such as maps and mapping, flannel boards, un-serialized posters, drawing and discussion, ranking, rating, sorting, and open-ended stories (Davis-Case 1989: 19). Besides identifying problems, the network or community should also discuss and list its own strengths and weaknesses in terms of level of health literacy of the members to use information relevant to health in the areas of healthcare, disease prevention, and health promotion; health, mental health, and well-being promotion; healthy living; behavioral change to tackle non-communicable and communicable diseases; quality of primary health care; information and surveillance capacity; ensuring safe basic commodities such as water, food, and sanitation; risks of a hazardous or contaminated environment; health-promoting social and environmental setting; level of media literacy of members; public health access, capacity, and effectiveness; and access to the internet, to mass media, telephones, and transportation (see more in *chapter 8*).

Samples of concrete examples of health behavioral problems, that a community together with a health communicator may need to take into consideration, are listed below:

Health Problems Related to Food Consumption

Health Problems Identified at the Individual Level

- Unable to read food labels. Do not understand how saturated fat, unsaturated fat, cholesterol, salt, sugar, additives, etc. have impact on health.
- Unable to choose a balanced diet. Nestle (2007: 77) advices:

  > "Eat less red meat. Eat less of high-fat dairy products. Eat a largely plant-based diet. Eat less red meat and less of fried foods, high-fat dairy foods, and processed foods. Eat foods low in fat, saturated fat, cholesterol, sugar, and salt."
- Forgot to check expiry dates on foods.
- Does not know how to cook. Have to rely on canned food and fast food.
- Does not know how to handle raw food hygienically.
- Does not know nutrition values of fresh food, frozen food, and canned food.

Health Problems Identified at the Organizational/Group Level

- Unable to participate in the promotion of low fat, low sugar, low salt diet.
- Is not aware of the correlation between soft drinks and fast food with obesity.
- Does not know how to share knowledge on food safety.
- Unable to be a watchdog on advertisements on foods and food supplements.
- Unable to participate in organic farming and co-ops.
- Does not support locally grown food.

Health Problems Identified at the Structural Level

- Does not know how to voice concerns to the government/authority to control and regulate advertisements on supplementary foods.
- Does not know how to advise the government/authority on control and regulate quality of seafood and meat.
- Does not know how to advocate for food labels enforcement and regulation.
- Does not know how to voice concerns on food advertisements.
- Does not know how to voice concerns on pesticides and insecticides in fresh vegetables and fruits, or hormones and antibiotics in meat and poultry, or the safety of fresh water fish and seafood.

Health Problems Related to Air-Borne Issues

Health Problems Identified at the Personal Level

- Cigarette smoke; smoke inside buildings or in public vehicles.
- Neglect to check car yearly so that it would not emit black exhausting fume.
- Neglect to have air-conditioners cleaned regularly to avoid legionnaire disease.
- Does not cover mouth when sneezing or coughing.
- Prefers to use automobile above public transportation and bicycle.

Health Problems Identified at the Organizational/Group Level

- Does not know how to voice concerns about smoking.
- Does not know how to approach government agencies to demand the enforcement of penalties on smoking in public space.
- Does not know how to request the implementation of governmental policies on the separation of residential areas from industrial or trading areas.
- Does not know how to advocate for biking lanes and underground subway systems.
- Does not know how to advocate for annual check-ups of vehicles.
- Does not know how to advocate for community air pollution monitoring.

Health Problems Related to Water-Borne Issues

Health Problems Identified at the Personal Level

- Does not drink filtered or boiled water.
- Drinks from hot plastic water bottles in a car.
- Re-use a plastic bottle for drinking.

Health Problems Identified at the Organizational/Group Level

- Does not know how to advocate for no trash in water ways.
- Does not know how to advocate for the control of contaminants in the water supply.
- Does not know how to advocate for no dumping of industrial waste in water ways.

Health Problems Identified at the Structural Level

- Does not know how to advocate for a clean water supply.
- Does not know how to advocate for the enforcement of penalties for trashing or dumping sewage or waste in waterways.

Health Problems Related to Medicine

Health Problems Identified at the Individual Level

- Does not complete the course of prescription drugs (especially antibiotics).
- Does not take prescribed medicine on time, such as daily for chronic disease patients.
- Uses medicine advertised in mass media and over-the-counter deliberately without consulting a pharmacist.
- Does not read labels or detailed explanation before taking the medicines.
- Does not know how to perform first aid at home.

Health Problems Identified at the Organizational/Group Level

- Does not know how to use medicine wisely.
- Does not know how to inform and explain about the correct way of using general medicines.
- Does not know how to advocate for first aid courses in the community.

Health Problems Identified at the Structural Level

- Does not know how to advocate for banning misleading advertising for medicine or health foods/supplements in the mass media.
- Does not know how to advocate for free primary healthcare.
- Does not know how to advocate for first aid course training in schools.

Types of Health Issues

To identify the right type of health issue, and select the appropriate advocacy communication strategy, Servaes and Malikhao (2010: 44) suggest the following distinctions within the world of health:

A Distinction at Level of Complexity of Health Problems

Let's take, for example, a communicable disease as malaria versus a cardiovascular disease. Malaria requires handling the problem of individual behavior vis-à-vis the risk of mosquito bites, but also attention to policies on access to both prevention (bed nets) and treatment, and ultimately and ideally malaria requires some attention given to the waters where mosquito breed. Cardiovascular diseases have more to do with lifestyles acquired over time, physical activity, smoking patterns, food patterns, etc. However, cardiovascular diseases will also require attention both to individual behaviors, policies and environmental factors. In other words, carefully tailored communication interventions emerge based on a profound understanding of the health problem encountered and at the same time drawn on the generic options about individual behavior, policies and environmental factors.

A Distinction at the Level of the Time-Frame for Health Problems

Emergency diseases as, for example, SARS or Swine Flu require very different communication responses compared to the long-term development-oriented health challenges, such as HIV/AIDS. Typically responses to emergency diseases become very vertical and mass media borne, containing high proportions of information dissemination and also social mobilization in response to the immediate needs that have emerged due to the emergency. The participatory approaches are seen in the form of social mobilization, and less as longer-term empowerment strategies. As for the long-term health challenges as HIV/AIDS, it contains both elements of urgency, due to the lethal dimension linked to each HIV transmission, but contains also strong elements of dealing with fundamental issues of poverty, gendered power imbalances, lack of voice of People Living with HIV/AIDS (PLWHA), issues of stigma and denial, etc. The differences in how to respond lay both in the speed of response, the way to organize the response, the way to make use of the media and also the content of the media program flow related to the health problem. Despite all the differences, in both long-term and short-term response, there is the need to deal with a mix of individual behavioral patterns, policy issue, and environmental factors. These are some of the common denominators in health communication.

A Distinction between a Broad-Based (Horizontal) Versus a Narrow-Based (Vertical) Definition of the Health Problem

A broader-based definition of the health problem would engage in a rights-based approach and move into issues of power and gender relations, socio-economic determinants of the problem and both collective and individually oriented responses. While the vertical approach focuses on one specific health problem, say tuberculosis, the horizontal approach entails a cross-cutting approach which may well tackle tuberculosis, HIV/AIDS, malaria and diabetes in one specific area. Communication-wise, the two different definitional approaches to a problem require each their strategic response, but both would ideally require some longer-term intervention.

Health Issues in the Community

In order to recognize and define the health problems and issues in a community, the following steps could be considered:

Mapping Health-Related Issues in the Community

Different kinds of map charts help people to understand health-related issues easier. Issues can range from limited numbers of public toilets, safe water supply, vaccination, or primary healthcare in developing countries; or a number of fresh foods suppliers in a decaying neighborhood, waiting hours in an emergency room in a hospital, a number of people who lack health insurance, or a number of stalls in schools that provide fresh and healthy food in developed countries. Tally charts can be used to collect data. Then, a pie chart or a map chart can be made.

Regular Opinion/Attitude Surveys

Questionnaires can be used to help collect attitudes towards the current health situation. Open-ended questionnaires can be used to probe the opinion of the stake holders. No less than 30 samples can be selected by systematic random sampling to ensure inferential statistical significance. A systematic random sampling will ensure that everyone in the community has a chance to be selected. This can be done by a draw. Simple data analysis can be done by just tallying or using EXCEL or SPSS or other statistical programs to help process the data.

(Mass) Media Content Analysis

Read or watch and categorize keywords from the content of the mass media that published or presented information about the particular health-related issues. See how it was covered and investigated, and key issues.

Also the analysis of communication-materials (newsletters, leaflets, video clips, websites, images, scripts for radio or theatre plays, etc.) is important. Read or watch and note down important clues and problems found in communication materials. See how each material covers the issue in-depth. Think of how you can change anything to make it better.

Networking

Systematic and continuous networking (both in real and virtual space) with NGOs, interest groups, scientific institutions, public health bureaus, health care providers, and other civic communities is important. In addition, Servaes and Malikhao (2010: 48) highlight the importance of media and communication and communication through other means, such as physical contacts in health advocacy:

> "Media must be activated to build public support and upward pressure for policy decisions. Interest groups must be involved and alliances established for reaching a common understanding and mobilizing society. This calls for networking with influential individuals and groups, political forces and public organizations, professional and academic institutions, religious and cause-oriented groups, business and industry. Public demand must be generated and citizens' movements activated to evoke a response from national leaders."

Regular briefings/interviews and meetings with interest and lobby groups are useful to ensure support and advocacy to policy makers.

3. Setting Goals and Objectives

Discuss the objectives of the project in a group meeting and try to establish community objectives, which may not be the same as those of the beneficiaries. Normally short-term goals should be quantifiable or measurable. That can be assessed by questionnaires, tally or observation. Medium- and long-term goals can be assessed qualitatively by either in-depth interviews, focus group discussion, observation, or participatory observation.

Defining Indicators of Achievement

Sustainability indicators should be defined and assessed. Servaes et al. (2012: 27-28) have outlined a framework for the assessment of sustainability in social change as explained in *chapter 5*. Davis-Case (1989: 26) suggests that other kinds of indicators, such as indicators of relevance, effort, efficiency, utilization, coverage, and quality could be taken into account as well. These indicators are just examples. The teamwork can define other indicators which they think suitable for the project.

4. Identifying Resources

Resources can be donors, budgets, staff of health communicators, local members, public health volunteers, public health specialists, health care providers, primary health care units, schools, library, media centers, etc.

After identifying which health problem the network or community wanted to tackle, group discussion would follow to plan for media strategies to advocate for policy design and decision-making aimed at ensuring political, social and legislative support for the health issue; or advocacy for policy implementation which requires intensive efforts for mobilizing social forces, individuals and groups for development actions.

Appropriate Health Strategies

Distinctions in type of health problems result in the need to define appropriate strategies. Servaes and Malikhao (2010: 44-45) recommend some consideration regarding strategy selection at several levels:

Level of Intervention

The strategic communication response may be defined in relation both to local community-based constituencies, but also to national fora of either ordinary people or decision-makers in parliament or government. Furthermore, and a rapidly growing phenomenon, the transnational, regional and often global response mechanisms are gaining growing attention. For example, there has in recent years been increased recognition of HIV/AIDS not only being defined as a local or national problem, but also requiring transnational response mechanisms, which have been developing over the last decade.

Thematic Emphasis of Intervention

This ranges from focus on individual behavioral determinants to a broader socioeconomic, cultural and political focus. If we take the example of polio, there has been a significant change in focus from the extensive vaccination campaigns, focusing on social mobilization in the late 1980s, to today's broader-based campaigns with strong advocacy components. Most often, however, many organizations remain focused on behavioral interventions, as can be seen from those lifestyle-related health problems such as Diabetes Type 2. In fact we need to also emphasize the processes of urbanization and the consequential changes it has upon everyday life. We should keep in mind that *food politics*, which is a special relationship between the agro and food industry, advertising industry lobbyists, and the government cannot be neglected. For instance, Nestle (2009: 332-4) reveals how the food industry entices their target groups to believe that sugary food is healthy food.

Content of Intervention

Strategic communication —as it is understood in BCC— is embedded in the logic of producing messages directed at passive target audiences comparable to hypodermic needle injections. However, as advocacy communication, participatory communication and communication for sustainable social change are becoming more popular, we are now witnessing a growing emphasis on the assumption of the active audience that engages in collective reflection and action.

Coordination of Interventions

Natural disasters and emergencies have demonstrated the need to design and implement region-wide strategies, which require strong communication components. The 2004 Tsunami showed a lack of cooperation both in the immediate emergency and the subsequent response. On the contrary, the international response to the recent dengue outbreaks showed technical supports and collaborating network of laboratories as well as case management, prevention, and control of each affected countries (WHO 2015 e). Also, several international initiatives have provided strategic guidance for global and regional responses to health challenges, e.g., infant feeding, HIV/AIDS, child health. However, the communication component within these regional and global strategies is often limited to dissemination efforts and lacks specificity on specific communication strategies. That is why the UN-agencies have agreed to what they call a "One Country" approach to development issues, with one agency (most often UNDP) in charge of the coordination and supervision of the implementation of projects in the same region or country (see Servaes 2007, or UNESCO 2007).

The Importance of Process- and Evidence-Based Intervention Strategies

There is an increased emphasis on moving from a uniform focus on *results* to an increased focus on *processes* of empowerment. While monitoring and evaluation approaches focuses on health outcomes and impact communication indicators remain essential to health communication interventions, a focus on process will provide deeper understanding of the nuances and particularities of development and health, especially those that remain embedded in cultural practices. Within HIV/AIDS communication it is seen in moving from a narrow focus on individual behaviors (for instance, the Abstinence, Be faithful and use a Condom—ABC model in HIV/AIDS prevention) to, for example, PANOS's document (2006) on how communication can support HIV social movements to achieve inclusive social change, or what role culture and religion can play in HIV/AIDS prevention campaigns (Malikhao 2007, 2008). In the latter cases the expected outcome is a process of empowerment. As a result, a focus on context and communities as units of analysis has emerged as critical to understand the effectiveness of interventions in health promotion and communication (Omoto 2005; Papa, Singhal & Papa 2006).

Health Communication Approaches

Last but not least, we would need to agree on whether to use communication alone or in a mix with other tools to communicate about/for health.

Communication as an Independent Instrument

One needs to decide if and when the group prefers to use a two-way communication process through various kinds of media to advocate changes on health issue; or whether a single top-down approach is considered more efficient to generate results in, for instance, a crisis situation.

Media Selection

Media selection depends on the media habits of the stakeholders or audiences. This can be found out through a focus group discussion together in combination with survey research. See *chapter 6* for media choices.

Message Design

The message should aim to suit the demographics of a community. Important criteria for the success of advocacy messages, reported by Servaes & Malikhao (2010: 48), are:

- Relevance: the issue has to be considered relevant to the several stakeholder groups;
- Timing: the issue has to be put on the agenda at the right time;
- Validity: the information and statistics provided have to be valid;
- Cultural sensitivity: the information should be tailored to the audiences and be in line with the understandings and expectations of people and stakeholders;
- Orientation of the relevant stakeholder groups: stakeholder groups have to be trained in interpreting data, so that they are able to understand them.
- Communication: interaction and reaching mutual understanding(s) between relevant stakeholder groups;
- Action orientation: advocacy strategies have to provide information for concrete action;
- Dissemination of information: advocacy messages and information can only be used by decision-makers if they are disseminated properly.

Keep in mind that information or messages are not knowledge. Knowledge is accumulated in the social memory in various forms such as myths, legends, stories, etc (Salas & Tillmann 2010: 12). Knowledge is socially constructed. What one person knows is not necessarily the same as what the other perceives. Each individual selects, retains, and (re)constructs information differently, depending on his/her experience and sociocultural differences (Sales & Tillmann 2010: 12). That's why messages need to be tailored in content and physical appearance according to the health issue and sociocultural factors, such as gender, age groups, and education levels. The teamwork needs to consider the combination of all possible actors and factors.

Messages for females should be geared towards their specific reproductive health problems, such as advocacy on breast cancer screening; for males that could be an antismoking campaign, or drink driving because males tend to smoke and drive faster than females. Messages for children should contain more graphics and the language used should be simple. Messages for the elderly group should use larger fonts for easy reading. Messages for the less educated should contain more graphics or should be in audio or video formats rather than in text.

Messages need to trigger people to action by offering a new loop of habit. Many messages that provide dietary guidelines do not actually change the people's eating behavior because they only 'inform' and do not suggest a new routine out of the fast food habit loop of routine-rewards, as explained in *Chapter 2*. The message would need to state a simple and obvious cue and clearly define the rewards. For instance, a cue of planned plant-based meal images for each day with the reward that it will be lower bad cholesterol levels (LDL) would be more effective.

Media Production

At this stage the teamwork should know which media they are going to use. A health communicator with media literacy or a facilitator who is specialized in media production can be useful to advise the team about how to prepare for media production. For videos and digital storytelling, a group discussing on a script and evaluating the script could be the starting point. Filming and editing can be done by group members. For a website, a webpage, or a blog, participatory decisions about the web design, content, and theme can be reached. For print media, artwork and content can be decided by the group. Print media can accompany the digital media with more in-depth information. However, keep in mind that they are for people with at least a basic level of literacy.

Informing Groups on the Use of Other Instruments (New Laws, Subsidies, Etc.)

Apart from the message design, a peer group or social support needs to be planned to keep people away from their old undesirable habits. Self-discipline and will power can be trained so that people have autonomy to make a determined cue to get into a habit loop with positive rewards to health behavior. School-based education is a good choice to foster desirable health behavior from a young age onwards. Hygiene; gender understanding; reproductive health; vaccinations against many communicable diseases such as Polio-Tetanus-Diphtheria vaccines and their effects, Human Papilloma Virus (HVP) vaccines, etc; healthful food selection and preparation; sex education; health- and media literacy can be put in a school curriculum.

Certain health issues should be addressed not only by mobilizing for behavioral changes of the stakeholders but also to influence the policy makers to make changes at a structural level. Therefore, legislation of laws or infrastructure changes can be useful to control the aspired health behavior up to a sustainable level.

Monitoring and Evaluation (M&E) through Qualitative Research

Participatory monitoring and evaluation is a tool to improve on the current project and plan better next time. Who will participate in an evaluation depends on the purposes of the evaluation; the process involves engaging stakeholders and any relevant actors in decision-making on M & E, designing the evaluation, selecting the indicators for M & E, collecting the data, analyzing the results and using the information for their own purposes (Karl 1999: 108, 115). Participatory methodologies and techniques, as adapted from Karl (1999: 115), are:

- Questionnaires and surveys
- Video conference
- Interviews of various stakeholders in the network
- Focus group discussions of different stakeholders or their representatives.
- Group review of data collected in monitoring of publications, reports, and other written materials. Website, blog, social networking page content evaluation.
- Observation or anecdotal evidence of the effects and impact of activities.
- Role playing.
- Team field visits.
- Group analysis and presentation of data.
- Mapping exercises of the field of work.
- Group analysis of case studies.

5. Maintaining Control of the Public Health Problem

The public health problem can be further discussed as public information via print media, websites, community radio, or community TV or other forms of community media. Information on changes of policy design and implementation can be shared via selected community media. Regular opinion/attitude surveys (since age-linked target groups will be replaced slowly by younger generations) provide a longitudinal perspective.

Communication as Part of a Social Media Network

Social media marketing strategies are similar to those of social marketing, but social media marketing has more advantages, thanks to advanced digital communication. Those advantages are, for instance, creating a buzz online that could promote our health-related messages; enabling the followers/users to promote the messages themselves; and encourage user participation and dialogues (Barker et al. 2013: 3). Advanced ICT makes participatory social marketing under the multiplicity paradigm possible. It is a low cost but effective strategy for health communication. (We already discussed social media for social marketing in *Chapter 5*).

Health communicators can get to the hearts of the millennials or younger generations by using this communication approach. Health communicators can host online discussions on health-related issues and build trust with the stakeholders. The participatory social marketing or social media for social marketing strategy, as adapted from Barker et al. (2013 26-27, 29, 94-95, 151), can be summarized as follows:

- Listening to what people are saying about health-related issues.
- Setting goals by checking the needs, behaviors, and tastes of the stakeholders. Conducting a survey or competitive analysis to determine the community strength

regarding health literacy, wellness, well-being, etc. Goals include community building, increase the wellness of community inhabitants, increasing awareness on health-related issues and diseases, improving perception on the community capacity, creating more positive impressions with the stakeholders regarding health care, expanding the engagement arena to include more people in the community, driving word-of-mouth recommendations for health communication, producing new ideas of promoting health, and generating leads, handling crisis management, and public relations to the media health communicators use.

- Determining strategies by categorizing the social media platforms in a community. Listening and learning how to behave. Engage stakeholders to participate in the social web. In this case a health communicator acts as a contributor, not a promotor. His/her role is to build up relationships and contribute content to build reputation and become a valued member of a community. Connect with everyone online and offline. Increase search engine ranking and site traffic.
- Identifying the members of the online community. Gather relevant demographic information.
- Selecting tools (new media choices are explained in *Chapter 6*). This can be done when finding the social media sites where the members reside and then focusing efforts on those platforms.
- Implementing. This is an integration of goals, strategies, audience, and tools. Publishing blogs need to use catchy titles, update frequently, keep posts concise and focused, invite comments, promote the blog by signing up with a popular blog listing service, and engage with others by making thoughtful comments and responding to other people's comments. Blog publishing demonstrates the writing skills and human relations skills of a health communicator.

  Publishing podcasts and webinars need to design content (preferably in a participatory fashion). Producing podcasts requires an articulate moderator, creating talking points, not reading scripts, brevity, avoid over-editing, and include music. Hosting webinars is relatively low cost. Listening and rhetoric skills are needed.

  Publishing articles online can be done on certain directories such as eHow.com, Squidoo.com, EzineArticles.com, etc.

  Sharing videos online is another way to engage discussion on a health-related topic. To share videos widely, one needs to pass through three stages of sharing: primary, secondary, and tertiary. Primary sharing is about posting it online for the first time. Secondary sharing occurs when early viewers spread the video within their own social circles. Tertiary sharing is when the content is spread on the Internet by people who do not know or have no connections with the original video's creator(s). In order to spur tertiary sharing, a health communicator needs to give each video a descriptive and memorable title, different titles, tags, keywords associated with the video on each online video sharing website. Encouraging others to share is part of user generated content (UGC) which is useful in a social media campaign. To produce a successful video, one must focus on content first. After the participatory production, the health communicator needs to promote the channel via either YouTube, blog posts, or other social networks. Update it frequently and keep up with the numbers of viewing and comments on content.

Sharing photos online, on Flickr, Photobucket, SmugMug, Shutterfly, SnapShot etc., allows online stakeholders to comment, rate and tag pictures. Images of the community, meetings, events, can be shared, commented, and exchanged. It is good publicity for a health communication campaign.

- Monitoring. This includes tracking, measuring, and evaluating the community social media for social marketing initiatives.
- Tuning to constant adjusting and improving the elements of the plan for improvement.

CONCLUSION

Sustainability in health is a national goal to engage and include every sector in the society: civil society; private and public institutions, such as public health, schools, hospitals; the media institutions, communities, and individuals. Leadership from the government at all levels, especially the public health ministry and public health agencies, is important to improve old or health policies or to issue a new one and ensure a smooth and transparent inter-sectoral collaboration. Good governance requires accountability, justice, fairness, and virtues to ensure health for all. Media and communication are necessary to empower all members of society to take health in their own hands and come up with concerns and advice to policy makers. Advocating or mobilizing health from a community upwards to the top health authority or half way to meet the top-down chains of disease prevention, health promotion, and surveillance ensures people-centered health systems and enriches community capacity and resilience to cope with challenges. Achieving good health for communities indicates good human-development capacity.

Health communication strategies presented in this chapter are guidelines for each community to come up with its own strategies. Communication for awareness, attitude and information on health issues has been discussed in many books but communication for health knowledge and health behavior is what the strength of this book and this chapter is about. It is possible to foster health behavior and transfer knowledge, but that cannot happen without the empowerment of the people in the community, regardless of gender, age, social status, education, and ethnicity or race.

REFERENCES

Barker, M., Barker, D., Bormann, N. & Neher, K. (2013). *Social Media Marketing. A Strategic Approach*. Australia: South-Western Cengage Learning.

Baum, F., MacDougall, C., & Smith, D. (2006). Participatory Action Research. In *J Epidemiol Community Health*., 60: 854-857. (Doi: 10.1136/jech.2004.028662).

Chan, M. (2013). Foreword. In *Health 2020. A European Policy Framework and Strategy for the 21st Century*. Cohenhagen: World Health Organization (WHO) Regional Office for Europe, p. 8.

Davis-Case, D. (1989). *Community Forestry. Participatory Assessment, Monitoring and Evaluation*. Rome: Food and Agriculture Organization of the United Nations.

Karl, M. (1999). Networks and Networking: Conclusions and Challenges. I. 1 Introduction. In M. Karl, A. Anand, F. Blankenberg, A. van den Ham, et al. (Eds.) *Measuring the Immeasurable. Planning Monitoring and Evaluation of Networks.* New Delhi: Women's Feature Service., pp. 17-26.

Nestle, M. (2007). *Food Politics. How the Food Industry Influences Nutrition and Health.* Berkeley-Los Angeles-London: University of California Press.

Nestle, M. (2009). *What to Eat.* New York: North Point Press.

Omoto, A. (2005). *Processes of Community Change and Social Action.* Mahwah: Lawrence Erlbaum Associates.

PANOS (2006). *Speaking Freely, Being Strong: HIV Social Movements, Communication and Inclusive Social Change.* London: The Panos Institute.

Papa, M., Singhal, A., & Papa, W. (2006). *Organizing for Social Change. A Dialectic Journey of Theory and Praxis.* New Delhi: Sage.

Servaes, J. (2007). Harnessing the UN System into a Common Approach on Communication for Development. *The International Communication Gazette,* Sage, 69, 6, pp. 483-507. (http://gaz.sagepub.com).

Servaes, J. & Malikhao, P. (2010). Advocacy Strategies for Health Communication. *Public Relations Review*, pp. 42-49. (Doi: 10.1016/j.pubrev.2009.08.017)

Servaes, J., Polk, E., Shi, S., Reilly, D. & Yukupitijage, T. (2012). Towards a Framework of Sustainability Indicators for 'Communication for Development and Social Change' Projects. *The International Communication Gazette,* pp. 1-25. (Doi: 10.1177/17480 48511432598).

UNESCO (2007). *Harnessing Communication to Achieve the Millennium Development Goals.* Paris: UNESCO.

World Health Organization Regional Office for Europe (2013). *A European Policy Framework and Strategy for the 21st Century.* Cohenhagen: World Health Organization (WHO) Regional Office for Europe.

Websites

World Health Organization (WHO) 2015
WHO 2015 e dengue and severe dengue
http://www.who.int/mediacentre/factsheets/fs117/en/, accessed on Jan 17th, 2016.

Chapter 8

HEALTH COMMUNICATION STRATEGIES FOR SUSTAINABILITY: HOW TO DO IT!

ABSTRACT

This chapter is a continuation from the previous chapter. Participatory-based communication strategies as bottom-up approaches will be the highlight of this chapter. They will be laid down step by step in as guidelines for health communicators, facilitators, public health specialists, and interested students and scholars to creatively mobilize (community) media and communication knowledge, skills, techniques, and technology to improve health through a life-course of empowering people; tackling local major health challenges of non-communicable diseases, injuries and violence, and communicable diseases; strengthening people-centered health systems, public health capacity and emergency preparedness, surveillance and response; and creating resilient communities and supportive environments. In addition, environmental impacts on health will be assessed, as well as risk communication in times of disasters and epidemics.

Keywords: empowerment, participatory-based media advocacy, participatory-based communication strategies, participatory-based mobilization strategies, people-centered health systems, resilient community, capacity building, emergency preparedness

INTRODUCTION

Continuing from the previous chapter, this chapter discusses in-depth participatory-based advocacy communication and communication for structural and social change strategies. Moreover, it provides practical examples for health communicators, public health specialists, educators, healthcare providers, etc. hoping that those interested can be inspired to create their own communication strategies to suit their communities.

To design communication strategies, a health communicator needs to be aware of the diversity of his/her audience, for instance the age groups, intellectual abilities, learning styles, educational levels, and cultural backgrounds. Communicating with teens or tweens, digital channels, graphics, and language used must be different from communicating with adults. Communication with people with intellectual disabilities may need more graphics and animation, and simplification of language. Computer-aided communication may be a good solution for people with different learning styles so that they can select a level of health education that suits them and to encourage them to learn at their own pace. Learning outside of a healthcare facility can occur at home. Websites that help stakeholders manage their weight, record daily exercise, etc. can be used for people with moderate media literacy. Cultural backgrounds should be considered when designing health promotion messages, such as food choices, healing beliefs, and exercise choices. Also the limitation of each media, e.g., the depth of the content, can be limited by the constraints built in each digital medium. For instance, Twitter is limited to140 characters per tweet. Instagram requires images and graphics. Certain health related websites help people manage their health issues with good feedback (Hayes & Aspray 2010: 44).

However, given the digital divide, not everyone can access information online. Some marginalized ethnic groups, or high risk groups or low income groups, have no access or little access to the internet. Health communicators should be able to strengthen human communication. S/he needs to see how s/he is going to make use of traditional media and personal media to their utmost capacity. Human relations are very important to change people's behaviors. One can be trained to give up old habits and replace that with new ones. That needs a supporting environment, such as a school-based intervention, a peer-to-peer communication, a support group, counseling, advice, moral support, etc. One can gain knowledge from information through social interactions. To reinforce a healthy behavior, we also need structural support by way of taxes, subsidies, law enactment, or law enforcement. Those are the challenges a health advocate or health mobilizer faces.

Being a facilitator, social advocate, or social mobilizer in a community, a health communicator should encourage online and offline participation in the following areas:

- Encourage the participatory-based creation of blogs, articles, videos, music, images, and art. Upload digital files to social media platforms. Send the materials to the mass media (newspapers, community media, local radio or TV station). Organize gatherings to show printed or video materials and discuss health issues with stakeholders.
- Upload and save digital favorites on bookmarking sites such as Delicious; share or tag photos on sites like Facebook and Flickr, and subscribe to RSS feeds to automatically receive new blog posts by the people in the community (virtual or physical). Help organize and categorize content on the social web (Barker, Barker, Bormann, and Neher 2013: 53-54).
- Collect pieces of information from newspapers, magazines, and journals on certain health issues and organize exhibitions for the people in the community. Inform about health news on community websites, community radio, blogs, microblogs as well as posters.
- Facilitate group discussions and conversations on social networks such as Twitter, Facebook, LinkedIn, and Eon, as well as facilitate group discussions and conversations on community radio, community TV and organized events.
- Support outreach and peer education activities by integrating community media, social media, and personal media.
- Evaluate and comment on content produced by creators and be a moderator in the community's discussion forums. Correct wiki articles.

- Co-ordinate and network with the government, public and private sector, NGOs and civil groups through phone calls, e-mails, text messaging, meetings, sharing videos, etc.

Texting on cell phones or tweeting can be used as a publicity strategy to introduce the media and content on health communication. Also, door-to-door knocking, telephone calls, mailing/leaving a leaflet in the mailbox, can be used to promote events, blogs, websites, meetings, seminars, and training courses. The media that can be considered are personal media, community media, and social media. Radio and theatre plays can be traditional media for people with low literacy rates. Blogging, creating a website, creating a webpage on social media, podcasting, and webinar can be alternatives for a digitally savvy community.

Health communication strategies proposed in this book are adapted from the four WHO strategies and action plans of the European regional and global levels (WHO Europe 2012: 69). Sustainability in health means that a longer life, a healthy lifestyle, healthy environment, good mental health, good people-centered health care, monitoring, control, prevention and treatment of diseases are expected in the long run. To achieve sustainability in health, communication strategies are one of the major contributing factors. These strategies concern:

1) Communicating strategies to improve health through a life-course of empowering people;
2) Communication strategies to tackle local major health challenges of non-communicable diseases, injuries and violence, and communicable diseases;
3) Communication strategies to strengthen people-centered health systems, public health capacity and emergency preparedness, surveillance and response; and
4) Communication strategies to create resilient communities and supportive environments, including a healthy physical environment.

1. Participatory-Based Media Advocacy and Mobilization Strategies for Improving Health through a Life-Course of Empowering People

Improving health through a life-course and empowering people requires multi-sectoral, both mixed top-down and bottom-up, communication approaches, and mixed media strategies to tackle health inequalities caused by gender discrimination, a hazardous environment, obesity and unhealthy lifestyles such as smoking or eating foods that have minimal nutritional values, globalization, and social change.

As advised by WHO Europe (2013: 73-74), our objectives should start with female-, infant-, child-, adolescent-, adult-, and the elderly health. Before we plan communication strategies we need to analyze our stakeholders. We could either check official demographic records of the community, or use a survey research method to have estimated population data of the stakeholders. In case of a community of interests or online community, we can send a survey online to find out about the attributes of our stakeholders. Then, a participatory process to identify issues related to improvement of health through a life-course and empowering people could start. Team members identify a cue, routine and reward for each health behavior such as breast feeding, eating nutritious food, monitoring a child's immunization rounds, etc. Then, they can plan for communication strategies. At this stage, it is assumed that health communicators are both health and media literates. A community radio, a community television, a community website and/or electronic mail could be used to send information and news to all members in the community.

Let's start with how to make women's health meet our sustainable goals. Health communication has been used to empower women in the areas of women's health status and child survival, including reproductive health, literacy, and education (Prasad 2009 b: 395-431). As women's health and reproductive health are essential for sustainable development, communication strategies which use community media should ensure that women receive professional care during antenatal, delivery, and postnatal stages by trained medical practitioners in a hygienic health institution. Mothers should be informed that they should breast feed their baby for the first six months of life; keep an immunization card for vaccination records of infants on BCG and Diptheria, Titanus, and Polio (DTP). They need to be aware of diseases of infants, such as diarrhea and vitamin A deficiency, have knowledge about nutrition, contraception, and reproductive health. At the same time, fathers should know how to take up parenting functions such as feeding, cleaning, playing, holding, showing affection, teaching, socializing, etc.

Women development means so much for the upbringing of their children. Empowering women to make their own decisions on their body and health is the first step. Next, women also need a good education, meaningful and safe jobs, and stable employment. All of these can be achieved if the government of each nation supports girls' education, equal chance to employment of females, child care and quality nursery, flexible working hours for the mother, maternal and paternal leaves with pay, and equal payment for a similar job as men. Discrimination against women, especially women from ethnic minorities, should be considered a crime.

Below are a few suggested participatory communication strategies for women's health for health advocates or health mobilizers:

Participatory-Based Communication Strategies for Women's Health

- Communication strategies aiming at an individual level

1) Promoting health- and media literacy to female stakeholders by providing a self-learning program online via a community website or inviting each individual to a training program. E-mails, snail mails, tweeting, phone calls, putting leaflets in mail boxes, posters at intersections, and text messaging on social media and on cell phones can be used to spread the news about the program online.
2) Promoting female education in public institutions, information on reproductive health, and the importance of infant first year of life by using folk media and community media. This is to raise awareness on women's issues. Podcasting, engaging discussions on social media, organizing webinars can be considered. Community radio and TV can provide a forum for discussion on this matter.
3) Promoting information on women's health and reproductive health on social media, community media, and the mass media. Videos on YouTube, links to websites on

this issue, podcasts, or vodcasts can be introduced on a community website or a web page on social media that a health communicator creates.

4) Promoting inclusion of women from other ethnic groups, who live in the community, by inviting them to participate in the production or activities of the women. Webinars and seminars can be organized. Video filming and vodcasting can be produced to embed them on a community website or webpage. Twitter and text messaging can be used to call for consultation, or sign up for webinars.
5) A health communicator sends (e-)mail to each pregnant woman who is registered for care at a health care institution so that they receive adequate information. Personalized reminders by post or by twitter, or text messaging or a phone call will be sent to remind the audience of vaccination or health check-ups due.
6) Using phone calls to make appointments for personal contacts with new mothers for the immunization of their infants. Home visits to new mothers can be arranged.
7) Having a health communicator and a practitioner visit each mother-to-be and new mothers regularly. Advise the mother-to-be on pre-natal and post-natal exercise/yoga classes, benefits of breastfeeding, supplementary medicines, nutrition, infant hygiene and clothes, and sleeping posture to prevent sudden infant death syndrome (SIDS). Encourage mothers to come to the healthcare center to weigh babies, and follow up on child development, etc. Discuss mental health of new mothers to prevent post-natal stress disorder. Listen to problems attentively and give advice.

- Communication strategies aiming at a group level

1) Training health care and medical personnel and interested stakeholders media literacy, communication and digital media skills. Posters, banners, brochures, a pdf file of tentative schedules sent via emails, public announcement via community radio or podcast, or a community broadcast tower, as well as promotion on a community website or webpage on social media, or a blog of the health communicator can be used to promote a training course.
2) Using community media such as community TV, video, or radio or website/webpage on social media, as well as podcasts to spread information and advice on breast-feeding, safe family planning, safe pregnancy and childbirth, including paternal assistance. Folk media such as street theatre or plays or songs can be used for edu-tainment.
3) Facilitating collaboration among families and other members in a community by producing participatory video clips or vodcasts on the importance of immunization, breast feeding, nutrition for mothers and babies, infant first aids – such as treating diarrhea or high fever before seeing a pediatrician. Non-violent ways of responsive care for babies and toddlers, emphasizing a warm and caring relationship in a family that fosters child mental, physical, and emotional health should be made and uploaded on community TV, vodcast, YouTube, community blog or website or a social media page (such as a Facebook page) devoted to health communication.
4) Organizing an event to invite and introduce all women to the community website; promoting links to clips on YouTube and on social media. Having personal contacts. Showing video clips that were participatory-produced and getting feedback.

5) Following up the event with a seminar or a webinar and discussion on relevant topics.
6) Forming a mothers' group online or offline to support one another with breast feeding and the autonomy to control reproduction. A blog would be appropriate to start with.
7) Raising awareness through participatory-producing podcasts, writing on social media and website, and organize events to raise funds to assist poor mothers from the less fortunate group.
8) Providing brain storming sessions with webinars or physical contacts for self-help groups to come up with cue, routine, and reward for building up healthy habits for women, especially mothers, such as eating more iron-rich and calcium-rich food during pregnancy, eat fresh fruit and vegetables, do aerobic exercises at least 30 minutes a day, drink enough water, etc. Film the sessions and upload video clips on the community website.
9) School-based intervention can be advocated to incorporate maternal and child health in a curriculum. Reproductive health and gender-sensitive education, emphasizing gender equality and non-violent ways of dealing with relationships, roles of mother and father in child development. This needs collaboration from schools and government officials.
10) Participatory evaluation of the media impact and program assessment for improvement.
11) Updating news, events, status on community websites, radio, and social networking pages regularly.
12) Maintaining relations and contacts with beneficiaries, both private and institutional ones. Also maintaining relations and contacts with politicians, leaders in the community, and government officials.

- Communication strategies aiming at a structural level

Forming women's groups and expanding the networks should be on top of the agenda. Contact politicians, government officials, and NGOs to draw their attention to women's issues. Show them the links, clips, and reports from the community. Virtual and offline group discussions on several issues, facilitated by health communicators, include:

1) Advocating for legislation to guarantee a women's right to her reproductive choices. Health communicators encourage and facilitate the production of video clips made by community members on a particular issue, and send the videos to public health authorities or write articles on websites, social networking pages, blogs, etc.
2) Advocating for the improvement of women education, including health- and media literacy, as well as advocating against female trafficking, or female exploitation in every possible way, by showing clips of interviewed women in the community and women training, or digital storytelling to be shown on diverse social media platforms or aired by community television and national channels.
3) Advocating for fairness and justice treatment towards women in terms of flexible working hours for those who have children, and quality day care for working mothers. Write blogs and reveal life stories of working women. Participatory videos

or vodcasts can be made with and about working women to be uploaded on YouTube or websites. Writing articles about these issues and have them published online, social media, or in the traditional mass media.

4) Advocating for attention to women's reproductive and child's first year of life health as the first year of life, while uploading participatory clips on YouTube and social media. Community media can be used to promote the clips. Events can be organized to promote a song for the first year of life with a PowerPoint presentation.
5) Advocating for inclusion of women from ethnic minorities and less fortunate women in education and work opportunities. This includes advocating for anti-discrimination laws against women and against women from ethnic minorities. Meetings and seminars or webinars can be organized. Stories and images can be uploaded on a dedicated website for women from ethnic minorities and on diverse social media platforms. Podcast and vodcast about the meetings can also be made.

Communication strategies for children and adolescent health will be discussed next.

Participatory-Based Communication Strategies for Children and Adolescent Health

Investing in the development of early childhood socially, emotionally, physically, and mentally would result in healthy and compassionate adults with maturity and a high moral standard. Discipline and good parenting are as important as good peers and the right context. Children need a safe outdoor environment to play and develop. Sports and extracurricular activities should be funded and supported by the community and school. Clean air, good water, good sanitation, and good housing guarantee a healthy living. Moreover, growing up in a stable family full of warmth and care, with both parents who have stable incomes and are educated, are important for childhood development. Religious and non-religious upbringing can yield a quality human resource if those emphasize positive thinking, humanity, social values, compassion, and good moral grounds. All these qualities are basic to any religion as principles for being good human beings. To be a sustainable human resource, one must be trained to be selfless and be concerned about one's physical, social and cultural environment. This can be achieved by applying the following participatory communication strategies for children and adolescent health:

- Communication strategies aiming at an individual level

1) Promoting useful links or *urls* that give information on gender equality on social media or youth websites.
2) Sharing links on a community website on how to delay sexual debuts. Forming a group of volunteer youth to educate and advice peers about STDs and HIV/AIDS on social media and offline.
3) Promoting the values of healthy lifestyles: eating fresh fruit and vegetables; aerobic exercises such as jogging, swimming, yoga, etc.; advocating for an alcohol-, smoke-, and drug-free life on new community media such as blogs, websites, podcast, digital

storytelling; community folk media, such as storytelling, theatre plays; community alternative media, such as posters, banners, news walls, etc.; community radio and community TV, social media, and the mass media.

4) Promoting health- and media literacy training programs. Campaigns can be initiated offline and online. Warn about the dangers of alcohol consumption and drug abuse. Twitter, text messaging, emails, public announcements on internet radio, local newspaper, community radio and TV can be good channels to publicize the programs. Collaboration with public authorities is important as well.
5) Promoting non-violent and non-discriminating ways to solve problems. Advocating compassion and loving-kindness in human relations.
6) Promoting inclusion of children and youth from ethnic minorities in the community.

- Communication strategies aiming at a group level

Media used can be personal media, community media, and social media.

1) Advocating for school-based comprehensive sex education for adolescents and adults in middle schools and colleges. Gender equality should be included in the curriculum. All kinds of contraceptive methods – such as pills, condom use, etc. --, HIV/AIDS prevention and other venereal disease prevention should be taught and discussed at school. This can be achieved by collaborating with schools, politicians, and official authorities. A participatory short film can be produced by a group of adolescents to be shown during meetings and uploaded on social media and community media networks. Also traditional community media, such as theatre plays, songs, and performances, can be used to send the gender equality message across.
2) Advocating for a school-based curriculum on media- and health literacy, and media- and health literacy courses in college. Strategies used can be similar to 1 above.
3) Facilitating training programs for media- and health literacy in the schools and colleges in a community. Strategies used can be as in 1.
4) Facilitating an intercultural communication program online via social media, community TV and radio, and training at schools and colleges in the community. Strategies used can be as in 1.
5) Facilitating participatory video clips promoting exercise, sports, eating healthy, gender equality, smoke-free, and alcohol-free lives. The clips can be uploaded on YouTube and other social media platforms or played on a community video player or included in a PowerPoint presentation for meetings and training purposes.
6) Facilitating participatory radio or television programs for children, tweens, and teens by letting all stakeholders in the community take part in the production process. The objective is to build up warm and caring families and communities.
7) Facilitate peer-to-peer education offline and online, and support groups on gender-responsive actions to discuss mental health, obesity, injuries, HIV and STDs, chronic diseases, sexual and reproductive health, violence and well-being. Promote these groups by organizing events. Podcast the content and post it on a weekly or biweekly basis. If it is a low-tech community, community radio or door-to-door visits and print media to promote these events should be fine.

8) Providing brainstorming sessions for self-help groups to come up with cue, routine, and rewards for building up healthy habits for children and adolescents, such as eating vegetables and fruit instead of fast food, learning how to cook a healthy and simple breakfast, exercise more, etc.
9) Facilitating teens and adolescent forums on healthy lifestyles, sex education, or disease prevention, on social media or mobile messaging applications such as LINE, WhatsApp, WeChat etc.
10) Organize fairs and events for children, teens, tweens, and adults in which community video products, exhibitions with posters, billboards, banners, and print media to promote a healthy lifestyle, health and counseling services are promoted to them.
11) Facilitating children and adolescents from disadvantaged families to produce participatory digital storytelling to advocate for a better livelihood, a better environment, and a good education.

- Communication strategies aiming at a structural level

Besides writing blogs and articles online, or using social media platforms or community media, one could send participatory-produced videos to the mass media or write to the media to draw the attention of local politicians in the community. Collaborating and networking with community leaders, authorities, NGOs, and civil groups is important. The following strategies could be considered:

1) Advocating for clean air, clean water, and safe housing by assessing the status of pollution.
2) Advocating for measures to control tobacco or alcohol use, or substance abuse.
3) Advocate to control and regulate advertisements for sugary foods and drinks, and foods high in trans-fatty acids, high saturated fat food, and salty food aimed at children and adolescents.
4) Use community media, print media, and personal contacts with policy makers and opinion leaders to advocate for safe playgrounds for children, sport fields, parks, and recreation space for children, youth, and families in the community.
5) Advocate for laws against cyber- and physical bullying.
6) Advocate for the inclusion of children and adolescents from ethnic minorities and less fortunate children.
7) Advocate for the participation of children and adolescents in environmental protection and on other awareness-raising social issues.
8) Advocating for a health information system for children and adolescents.

Next, adult health will be discussed. Career and employment, family life, work-life balance, taking care of aging parents, healthy lifestyles, safe work environments, stress and substance abuse, and childhood upbringing, level of education, social status, and many more, are contributing factors to adult physical and mental health. In this age group, people are prone to develop non-communicable diseases. Reflecting on a healthy lifestyle is a good way to start:

Participatory-Based Communication Strategies for Adult Health

- Communication strategies aiming at an individual level

New media, community media, social media and mass media can be used in an integrated fashion.

1) Promote a healthy lifestyle, a life free from alcohol and substance abuse, by sharing videos and digital stories on social media, podcasting, community radio and TV programs. Also writing in community newspapers, organizing community forums and other events can be considered to enable people to take informed decisions about their health and treatment in time of sickness and illness, and to monitor the quality of healthcare services.
2) Promote a healthy sex education and create awareness about STD and HIV/AIDS prevention (by sending health news via personalized e-mails).
3) Promote health education on communicable and non-communicable disease prevention and treatment. Apart from print media, video sharing, podcasts, community media can be considered. Collaboration with public health specialists and health care providers to organize an event for this purpose. Film the event and upload the video on YouTube. Post the link to social media and on the community webpage.
4) Promote benefits of living in good and clean housing, settings, and environment. In tropical zones, inform about the dangers of rodents and mosquitos. Video sharing, photo sharing via social media, as well as mobile exhibitions with video and digital stories can be considered.
5) Promote health literacy and media literacy by organizing a training program for participants. Social media, phone calls, public announcements via community radio, TV, emails, text messaging to raise awareness of the training program.
6) Promote rights, fairness, and justice for women via the mass media, community media, and social media. Sharing good videos, articles, and digital storytelling clips via appropriate channels. Offer free subscription to messages from health communicators.
7) Promote health education for families honing at parenting skills. Same strategies as in 6 can be considered for young parents. Collaborate with schools to organize meetings with parents. Follow-ups can be done via the community or school websites.
8) Personal media can help unlearn old habits of eating fast food, smoking, consuming sugary drinks and snacks, and staying idle, to be replaced with new habits of eating fresh vegetables, whole grains, fruit, exercise and control diet. A workshop can be organized and followed up with online or offline discussions.
9) Promote rights for preventive information against diseases, and for patients to receive proper and useful information.

- Communication strategies aiming at a group level

1) Produce participatory video clips on a healthy lifestyle for adults. Upload them on YouTube; post them on social media; post them on the community website, on electronic community media, and in print media.
2) Organize a training program on media- and health literacy for adults and parents. Develop digital stories to advocate for the importance of media- and health literacy.
3) Organize an online or offline support group to enhance skills for the re-employment of unemployed long-term adults.
4) Organize peer-to-peer online or offline exchanges on mental health-related issues, taking care of the elderly and the disabled, or cessation of discrimination against women, the elderly, ethnic minorities on employment opportunities.
5) Organize an online or offline group on alcohol and substance abuse among adults.
6) Organize a support group to monitor communicable diseases or environmental problems that affect health risks in the community. Mobile technologies can be used to share information and photos on social media.
7) Produce programs on community media to promote eating vegetables and fruit, exercising more, or how to stop smoking or substance abuse. Share clips, information, and images via social media networks.
8) Organize brainstorming sessions for self-help groups online or offline to build up healthy habits for adults, such as never to skip breakfast in the morning, exercise more, etc.

- Communication strategies aiming at a structural level

Besides writing blogs and articles online, or using social media platforms or community media, one could send participatory-produced videos to the mass media or write to the media to draw the attention of local politicians in the community. Collaborating and networking with community leaders, authorities, NGOs, and civil groups is important. The following strategies could be considered:

1) Advocate for equal opportunities for women and man. Organize a media campaign to raise this issue upward to policy makers.
2) Advocate for the inclusion of ethnic minorities, unemployed, and other marginalized groups to promote intercultural communication skills on community media programs.
3) Advocate for companies to offer a safe work place environment and to provide good occupational health services.
4) Advocate via personal contacts, organizing an event, uploading of videos on YouTube and other social media platforms for the inclusion of the unemployed and other high-risk groups in developing tools for risk management.
5) Advocate for clean air, safe water, and adequate sanitation; in other words, for a green and clean environment.
6) Produce a video clip to advocate on quality healthcare and counseling services with volunteers to help the elderly and the disabled, the marginalized, and other disadvantaged groups.

7) Advocate for recreation spaces, parks, sport fields, swimming pools for the public, and fitness centers in companies.
8) Advocate for a civic society where patients can be involved at all levels. Inviting debate about social welfare and protection, health and health care.
9) Advocate for legal rights for patients, provisions of professional liability, redress, and compensation in case patients are harmed.
10) Advocate for regulating and monitoring tobacco and alcohol consumption.

The next stage of life is the elderly phase. Quality of life in this phase gives the elderly a chance to participate in the community and pass on good experiences to the younger generation. In other words, to age with dignity, without any economic burden from medical costs and hospitalization to the government or family.

Participatory-Based Communication Strategies for Elderly Health

It is said that the elderly are not savvy on social or new media. That may be changing. However, traditional mass media, such as print media, radio, and television continue to be more preferred and should therefore be considered as strategic tools. A combination of various community media and personal contacts would work best for the elderly.

- Communication strategies aiming at an individual level

1) Promote media- and health literacy to the elderly in the community by organizing free training classes. Phone calls, snail mails, and e-mails can be the channels for contacts.
2) Promote a healthy lifestyle (exercise, eating right, and rest well) through online media, community media, and mass media. Home visits are important. Use personal media to contact the elderly, and listen to their stories/problems.
3) Raise awareness and provide information about routine immunization programs for the elderly, such as seasonal influenza shots.
4) Raise awareness on dementia prevention and other mental health disorders, such as anxiety and depression.

- Communication strategies aiming at a group level

1) Organize a training course on health literacy for the elderly in the community media.
2) Produce video clips to promote a healthy life style for the elderly.
3) Empower the stakeholders to organize peer-to-peer advice and support groups on mental health and domestic problems.
4) Promote the inclusion of the elderly in community events.
5) Advocate for the provision of classes in a community, such as ballroom dancing, tango, yoga, singing lessons, and other hobbies.

- Communication strategies aiming at a structural level

Media selection is more or less the same as those for adult health. The following strategies could be considered:

1) Advocate for legal and financial support for poor seniors.
2) Advocate for the reduction of fees for prevention and treatment for the elderly.
3) Advocate for a healthcare unit for elderly health in each community.
4) Advocate for online facilities for the elderly in public libraries.
5) Advocate for a hobby room or a club for the elderly in a community center.
6) Advocate for an outdoor and indoor meeting space for the elderly in a community.
7) Advocate for events that include the elderly to honor their experiences and expertise.
8) Advocate for community outreach to the elderly who are in need of help, and contact the appropriate NGOs, foundations, and authorities.

2. Participatory-Based Media Advocacy and Mobilization Strategies to Tackle Non-Communicable Diseases, Injuries and Violence, and Communicable Diseases

Participatory-Based Communication Strategies to Tackle Non-Communicable Diseases (NCDs), Injuries and Violence

Non-communicable diseases can, according to WHO Europe (2013: 92), be categorized into three groups: cardiovascular diseases, cancer, and mental disorders. They manifest as a complex intervention of risk factors, underlying determinants, and opportunities along the life-course and the course of a disease. Communication strategies to prevent these diseases should promote a healthy life style, disease prevention, active access to high risk groups, effective treatment and care, and integrate policy and action to achieve health equity. The mass media, social media, community media, as well as portable mobile devices can be used in an integrated fashion together with personal media.

- Communication strategies aiming at an individual level

Participatory-based social marketing via social media can be used to reach the stakeholders, who are mostly adults of more than 45 years old. Participatory-based video clips, mp3 files, can be made to inform and raise awareness on how to prevent NCDs. The most important strategies for edutainment include:

1) Promote healthy eating habits and work out regularly. According to Israpisit M.D. (Wellness city.co.th 2015), eat well, rest well and exercise, are the keys for individual prevention. He explains ten rules to fight NCDs consisting of five don't's and five do's. First of the don't's is do not foster negative thinking; maintain a clear mind. Second, do lose weight when you are overweight. Third, do not eat granulated sugar. Fourth, do not eat transfats; replace transfatty acids in food with

polyunsaturated fat. Fifth, do not eat mammal meat—such as pork or beef – because they have the same biochemistry as humans. This sort of meat is hard to digest and it will remain in our digestive system for three days. Poultry and fish are recommended. Five do's are recommended: first, eat fresh fruits and vegetables and reduce salt consumption. Eat non-sweet fresh fruits (preferably green fruit) for half of your appetite first (a green fruit has less sugar than a ripe fruit), and eat then your main meal, which should contain a large amount of raw fresh vegetables. Ripe fruits can be eaten after meal so that the sugar from the fruit comes to the blood streams slowly, because it blends with residue fibers from the meal. Second, eat whole grains in small amounts according to your age. The older one becomes, the smaller the amount of whole grains one should consume. Third, exercise at least 30 minutes daily. Preferably brisk walking. Fourth, sleep at least four hours a day and go to bed around 10 pm because the growth hormone in our body is excreted at night between 10 pm and 2 am to repair the damage cells while we are sleeping. Fifth, foster positive thinking and imagination.

2) Promote the afore-mentioned life-course strategies as the onset of non-communicable diseases, such as type 2 diabetes mellitus and heart disease, begin in early fetal life (WHO Europe 2013: 89).
3) Stress the importance of getting an education, as a higher education status is associated with healthier eating and less smoking (WHO Europe 2013: 89).
4) Raise awareness of monitoring the Body Mass Index (BMI – which is calculated from the height and weight of adults) so that it stays between 18.5-24.9, blood sugar, cholesterol, and blood pressure.
5) Raise awareness and give information on vaccinations against hepatitis B (to reduce the chance of liver cancer) and human papillomavirus (to reduce the chance of cervical cancer).
6) Promote the cessation of smoking and reduction of the amount of alcohol consumption.
7) Inform on palliative (end-of-life) care by sharing links to video clips and information.
8) Provide factual information on mental disorders, such as depression and anxiety. Reduce the discrimination towards people who live with mental disorders. Explain dementia in the elderly.
9) Encourage informed decision-making regarding non-communication disease treatment and mental health care.
10) Empower for non-violent ways of human relations and gender respect.
11) Engage stakeholders to take part in obeying traffic rules by encouraging them to report and monitor traffic rule violators.

- Communication strategies aiming at a group level

Participatory script writing for community radio or video production can be used to empower stakeholders to take NCDs, violence and injury issues in their own hands.

1) Empower the stakeholders to form peer-to-peer and support groups on refraining from tobacco use, drug misuse, and alcohol consumption.

2) Advocate for exercise and health promotion in the workplace. This needs collaboration among private business owners, public officials, and civil society at large.
3) Advocate for the establishment of a human rights group for non-communicable disease prevention.
4) Advocating for primary health care units that diagnose, assess, and assist with the management of non-communicable diseases. This needs good collaboration with public health, official institutions, and civil society.
5) Empower for first aids courses at the work place, in schools, and in the community.
6) School-based training on non-communicable diseases should be promoted to enhance understanding and promote healthy living.

- Communication strategies aiming at a structural level

1) Advocate for poverty deprivation to reduce mental health problems by establishing links among many sectors – education, public health, health care services, benefit offices, debt counsellors, and community mental health services. Personal media and participatory video clips or digital stories are very good to generate support from policy makers.
2) Advocate for the reduction of salt, sugar, and saturated fat in processed food of the food industry. This can be done in collaboration with MPs, authorities, civil groups, and consumer groups to the lobby for consumers' rights to healthier food legislation.
3) Advocate for monitoring and control of pesticides and insecticides used in fresh produce; and chemicals in meat, poultry, fresh water fish, and seafood. Networking with environmental groups, public health bureaus, agricultural sectors, MPs, community leaders, and consumer groups should push for legislation to control toxicity in fresh produce, meat, poultry, fresh water fish, and seafood.
4) Advocate for enforcements on pollution control for the industry and vehicles, for a safer and cleaner environment.
5) Advocate for stronger penalties for gender-based violence and sexual harassment at work.
6) Advocate for enforcement and heavy penalties for traffic rule violations to prevent accidents and injuries.
7) Advocate for heavy taxation on tobacco and alcoholic drinks.
8) Advocate for patients' rights to know about their treatment, and to be properly informed about the treatment procedure and medication.

Participatory-Based Communication Strategies to Tackle Communicable Diseases

Common communicable diseases found in both developing and developed worlds are, for instance, measles, mumps, and rubella; diphtheria, tetanus (also known as lockjaw), Acellular Pertussis (also known as whooping cough), poliomyelitis; HIV infection; TB and malaria; dengue and Severe Dengue fever; respiratory syndromes aggravated by crossings between the human virus and a virus normally found in animals, such as SARS (Severe Acute Respiratory Syndrome), which is also found in Himalyan palm civets (*Paguma larvata*) and raccoon dogs (*Nyctereutes procyonoides*) (Li et al. 2006), H1N1 or swine flu, H1N5 or Avian flu, MERS (Middle East Respiratory syndrome or camel flu); and hepatitis B and C. Participatory-based communication strategies require personal media, various community media, mass media and social media for social marketing.

Therefore, communicable diseases for which participatory-based communication strategies could be applied can be categorized into two different groups: vaccine preventable diseases and not-yet-available-of-vaccine preventable diseases.

To Tackle Vaccine-Preventable Communicable Diseases

- Communication strategies aiming at an individual level

1) Mass communication and various community media can be used for awareness campaigns for childhood vaccination and routine immunization for the elderly. Social media can be used for social marketing. Participatory-based social marketing is preferred in a community to create a preventive sphere. Personalized follow-ups for a second or third vaccination (if needed) should be done by phone calls, e-mails, text messaging, or snail mails. Personal media (such as nurses, public health specialists, midwives) are important for these follow-ups.
2) Links to information on vaccine-preventable communicable diseases should be shared online, either on websites or on social media platforms. Print media, such as brochures and small booklets, can be useful at primary healthcare units. Participatory video clips, to tailor towards most frequent vaccine preventable communicable diseases found in a community, should be shown at primary health care sites, community video points, community television, or a community website. It can be uploaded on social media platforms.
3) Provide links, and share information in the social media to seed discussions to enhance knowledge on the new development of vaccines, such as pneumococcal and rotavirus vaccines. Also, vaccines that bridge communication and non-communicable diseases, such as vaccine against hepatitis B and human papillomavirus,can be included.

- Communication strategies aiming at a group level

Advocate for the development of a surveillance and early-warning system in a community to monitor outbreaks of diseases by lobbying and showing participatory video clips to advocate for this purpose.

- Communication strategies aiming at a structural level

1) Advocate to collaborate via electronic means, telecommunication, and personal contacts with international organizations on sharing vaccine preventable

epidemiological data, laboratory-related data, evident-based and cost-effective interventions, etc.

2) Mobilize for social support for integrated collaboration across sectors. Law enforcement for childhood vaccination, subsidies for vaccination, poverty deprivation plans, employment opportunities, sanitation, hygiene, clean housing and public space, food and water safety.

To Tackle Not-Yet-Available and Non-Vaccine Preventable Communicable Diseases

Some important communicable diseases to be addressed respectively are malaria, TB, HIV/AIDS, and respiratory syndromes.

Malaria and Dengue Fever and Its Derivatives

- Communication strategies aiming at an individual level

1) Advocate via social media and community media to emphasize the importance of having bed nets against insects and mosquitoes, or mosquito and insect screens, on windows in residences in a hot and humid climate.
2) Empower via personal media and community media campaigns to monitor water puddles wherein mosquitoes can lay eggs around the neighborhood in a tropical zone.
3) Post and share information about disease transmission, symptoms, prevention, and the possibility of no treatments on community new media or social media to warn for the danger of people who have Dengue fever for the second time in life. Personal media, such as nurses or public health specialists, could be helpful in the discussion as well.
4) Encourage stakeholders to use or follow a training course on how to make biological/ organic mosquito and insect repellants to prevent insecticide resistant development of the virus that mosquitoes transfer. Video clips of how to make one's own repellant can be shown on community video points, community television, website or shared on YouTube. Twitter or text messaging can be used to promote the course.

- Communication strategies aiming at a group level

1) Advocate for an early-warning and surveillance system for Malaria and Dengue in a community. New cases can be shared among the data sharing networks.
2) Use participatory short film or video to advocate the government for inter-sectoral cooperation and raise funds or provide a budget for bed nets to the have-nots in a community, or a class training on how to make one's own biological repellant.
3) Empower the community dwellers to take the mosquito-free environment in their own hands via home visits, community radio, and social media.

- Cmuomnication strategies aiming at a structural level

Use participatory short films or videos to gain the inter-sectoral support and:

1) Advocate for a health information system that collaborates with other countries in sharing data and cases on Malaria and Dengue fever, and its drug resistant capability.
2) Advocate eradicating poverty by collaborating with civil groups, governments, private and public sectors.
3) Mobilize social support for the right of treatment and the right to have informed consent for Malaria and Dengue diagnosis and treatment.
4) Mobilize social support to upgrade poor living conditions.

Tuberculosis (TB)

- Communication strategies aiming at an individual level

1) Use the mass media, community media, and social media to inform stakeholders about the transmission of TB, symptoms, treatment, and prevention.
2) Participatory script writing for radio or podcast to provide information on TB drug resistance.

- Communication strategies aiming at a group level

1) Use social media to advocate the launch of a support and self-help group for TB.
2) Share appropriate videos on social media about the right of TB patients to advocate informed consent to treatments.
3) Use the media to advocate reaching out to a group of the people living with HIV, because this group has a high likelihood to develop TB. Personal media can be effective to empower them to TB prevention. E-mails and phone calls can be used to follow up. Social media can be used for discussion and consultation.

- Communication strategies aiming at a structural level

Use participatory video or digital stories in a community to advocate governments, public and private sectors, and civil groups. Good relations with key actors and politicians or MPs should be considered.

1) Mobilize social support for a health-information system for TB.
2) Mobilize social support to responsive health care services for TB diagnosis and skin testing, prevention, and treatment in the long run by using a comprehensive and participatory approach.
3) Mobilize social support for alcohol control, improving housing standards, and poverty deprivation, as high risk groups of TB are related to incarcerated people, alcoholics and homeless people (WHO Europe 2013: 100).
4) Mobilize social support for the right of treatment and the right to have informed consent for TB diagnosis and treatment.

HIV/AIDS

- Communication strategies aiming at an individual level

1) Participatory videos can be produced and watched to engage individuals to discuss how to collaborate within a community on HIV prevention and reduce discrimination against people who live with HIV/AIDS (PLWHA).
2) Participatory videos, digital storytelling, podcasts, and vodcasts can be uploaded to promote the importance of getting better education, as education increases the chances to a better occupation. HIV infection is related to poverty and a low socioeconomic status.
3) Promote digital storytelling clips to campaign on HIV transmission, HIV with alcohol, drug, and injection. Show how to make clean needles. Inform what kinds of sex risks spreading HIV (Granich and Mermin 1999: 45). Inform how to use condoms the correct way. Inform about the relationship between STD and HIV; and HIV and TB.
4) Promote via participatory community media the importance of anonymous HIV counseling and testing, especially to pregnant women.
5) Use personal media to train and organize home care for relatives of people living with HIV/AIDS (PLWHA).

- Communication strategies aiming at a group level

1) Use personal media and community media to advocate social support to care for people who are ill to prevent the spread of HIV. Use role plays, brainstorming, pictures to start a discussion, train and empower.
2) Use mass media, social media, and community media for social marketing on stop discriminating against people living with HIV/AIDS. Use personal media to engage the community with activities that include PLWHA as human resources.
3) Communities should be empowered to support outreach and peer education activities by using personal media together with community media. Social media for social marketing can be used to raise awareness.
4) Cultural values of communities must play a central role in changing HIV risk-taking behaviors and to encourage condom use.
5) Evaluation of community-based communication programs to prevent HIV/AIDS should be undertaken to improve on them.

- Communication strategies aiming at a structural level

1) Use the mass media to gain social support to promote HIV/AIDS prevention in sex education curricula at school. Gender education should be taught in such a way that it invites discussion, role plays, and brainstorming to emphasize gender-relevant knowledge and appreciation of women's roles, and indicate how violence towards females can be related to HIV infection.

2) Use participatory media to gain social support to assist women in rural areas with opportunities in education and technical training.
3) Use the media to gain social support on legislation against the discrimination of women by verbal abuse or behavior. Sexual harassment, sexual abuses, such as assaults and rapes, and female trafficking should result in high penalties.
4) Use the media to gain social support on legislation of laws and the enforcement of the law on alcohol misuse and drunk driving, drug and substance abuse, etc.
5) Use mass media to gain social support on comprehensive HIV prevention, such as providing clean syringes, promoting condom use, promote safer sex, and peer group education.
6) Use participatory media to promote a political environment that takes the public opinion into account in the policy-making process (for instance, access to antiretroviral therapy for people living with HIV/AIDS, employment for people living with HIV), and promotes a well-informed civil society and non-governmental bodies (UNAIDS 1999: 32).
7) Use integrated media to promote the linkage and integration of national programs on HIV/AIDS prevention with broader health and development agendas (WHO Europe 2013: 102).

Respiratory Diseases such as SARS, MERS, H1N1, and H1N5

Outbreaks and epidemics need to use risk management and a top-down approach to cope with the degree of severity and the coverage of the diseases. A participatory approach can complement the sustainability of risk management. Participatory films, clips, photos, or audio files can be used to integrate campaigns to engage the people and empower the community to strengthen their own capacity to tackle these diseases.

- Communication strategies aiming at an individual level

1) Use the mass media and community media to use social marketing strategies to inform senior citizens about flu vaccines. Personal media encourage them to register for flu vaccine shots.
2) Use social marketing, both mass and social media, to inform the community dwellers about the symptoms of diseases and the outbreaks, and advise them to wear a protective mask in times of an epidemic.
3) Use participatory media to help build up cleanliness, orderliness, and hygiene in households. Sanitary standards must be controlled regularly.

- Communication strategies aiming at a group level

1) Provide the healthcare workers with training courses to recognize the symptoms of respiratory diseases.
2) Use internal communication channels to promote quality assurance in a healthcare service place to make sure that the healthcare providers watch carefully for the possibility of antibiotic resistance. In concert with the internal communication,

community media can be used to advocate quality assurance in the healthcare service.

3) Use social media, community media, and the mass media to raise awareness in a group of seniors about the transmission and outbreaks of these diseases.
4) Use community media and social media to engage community dwellers in dialogues of how to perform risk management in times of epidemic outbreaks.
5) Use school-based interventions to teach students about hygiene, respiratory diseases, symptoms, prevention, orderliness and cleanliness.

- Communication strategies aiming at a structural level

1) Integrate participatory social media marketing with mass media convergence to gain social support, raise awareness and control the importation of respiratory diseases.
2) The participatory media can assist to improve laboratory data, epidemiological data, and evidence-based cases, and share them with other communities and countries.
3) Use participatory films, clips, photos, or audio files to mobilize social support for subsidies for flu vaccines for the underserved and senior citizens, and to improve housing standards.

3. Communication Strategies to Strengthen People-Centered Health Systems, Public Health Capacity and Emergency Preparedness, Surveillance and Response

People-centered healthcare means empowering the people to participate in decision-making about their own healthcare management and plan. This implies providing the people with access to adequate information about diseases, treatments, and rights, and cost effectiveness (WHO Europe 2013: 112). A selection of the most important participatory-based communication strategies are the following:

- Communication strategies aiming at an individual level

1) Participatory films, clips, or audio files can be used to advocate access and services for people with chronic diseases, with disabilities, and the aging group.
2) Participatory films, clips, or audio by healthcare professionals can be used to advocate for better working environments, flexible working arrangements, management support, and to gain social recognition.
3) The above media can be used to engage healthcare professionals in dialogues in training courses to enhance skills, decision-making, cultural and fiscal competencies.
4) The above-mentioned media can be used to address obesity, health inequality, and climate change to alert and engage the stakeholders with dialogues to come up with public health plans and strategies.
5) The above-mentioned media, together with personal media, can empower the stakeholders to participate in the design, implementation, and evaluation of health

policies and services. This includes mobilizing the social support for shared decision-making training between healthcare providers and patients.

6) Integrated participatory media can empower patients to make an informed decision about their treatments and rights.

- Communication strategies aiming at a group level

1) Use community media and participatory media to advocate for primary healthcare quality. Primary healthcare is important to promoting health behaviors and disease prevention. Media should inform the public about good links to primary healthcare and higher levels of care.
2) Media produced by healthcare professionals together with patients and people in the community can be used to advocate for good governance and alliances with other healthcare service places, engage the community to help design healthcare solutions, and ensure the quality of people-centered healthcare.
3) Meetings and dialogues with all actors and stakeholders involved will yield measures to assess the best people-centered health care service, and to discuss indicators for success.
4) Participatory media can be used to mobilize social support for good governance necessary for emergency preparedness and timely response to epidemics.

- Communication strategies aiming at a structural level

1) Using integrated participatory media together with the mass media to advocate for national strategies for developing public health services, revisiting current public health laws, reforming the laws if necessary, and reviewing ineffective partnerships.
2) Using participatory media to mobilize the public, private, and civil sectors to improve on structures and activities necessary to fight non-communicable diseases.
3) Using the afore-mentioned media to mobilize the stakeholders (public health workers, health care providers, patients, and the public) to seek ways of funding to cope with the cost of human resources, equipment, and medicines.
4) A long term planning approach depends on good governance and the engagement of all actors and stakeholders. Participatory media are good tools to gain social support for capacity building and appraisals of organizational performance to achieve international standards while sharing data and networking with accredited organizations abroad.

4. Communication Strategies to Create Resilient Communities and Supportive Environments, Including a Healthy Physical Environment

This topic requires a higher level of structural intervention (WHO Europe 2013: 123-127). Community-based media, especially participatory media, can be very helpful to advocate and mobilize efforts to develop and maintain sustainability in health and health for all. Environmental-associated diseases need collaboration from all sectors: private, public, civil, and governments. However, the level of strategies can be as follows:

- Communication strategies aiming at an individual level

1) Empower individuals to collaborate in the environmental management of their community by setting up a committee and a discussion online or offline forum to engage everyone.
2) Empower individuals to be citizen journalists to report and express concerns about water-borne, food-borne, air-borne, and zoonic-related outbreaks of diseases and extreme weather, by offering channels to share video clips, discuss problems, and solutions.
3) Empower individuals to monitor climate change and conserve the forrest/woods/ public ponds, canal and rivers, and air quality. Any kind of pollution should be reported by any community dweller. Any activities that contribute to the reduction of greenhouse-gas emissions should be supported.
4) Empower individuals to work out, use bicycles, recycle, and separate garbage.
5) Address and engage community dwellers to learn about types of garbage, and train everyone to separate and put garbage in the bin.
6) The media can be used to discourage community dwellers to burn wood or garbage by themselves.

- Communication strategies aiming at a group level

1) Create peer education and groups to discuss ways to help improve the environment.
2) Ensure public health so that everyone has access to safe water and sanitation.
3) Address obesity and injuries by training about safety in the house and a healthy diet.
4) Address and promote the importance of surveillance and preparedness systems for extreme weather events and disease outbreaks.
5) Create events to engage participation with community people, as well as school-based education to let the participants see the importance of recycling and garbage separation and not littering.
6) The media can be used to introduce new sources of clean energy, such as solar and wind energy.

- Communication strategies aiming at a structural level

1) Participatory media can be used to gain social support on measures, policies, and strategies to mitigate climate change.
2) The above-mentioned media can be used to mobilize social support on educational and public awareness programs regarding the environment and climate change.
3) The above-mentioned media can be used to mobilize social support for engaging the health sector and to control greenhouse gas emissions.
4) The media can be used to mobilize support for research and development on environmental conservation and climate change monitoring.

5) The media can be used to strengthen health, social welfare, and environmental systems and services to respond to climate change promptly.
6) The media can be used to redress the values of showing off material possessions, and to encourage people to use public transport and see the importance of urban planning, green and clean neighborhoods, and recreation spaces.
7) The media can be used to advocate for organized dumpsters that allow citizens to separate wastes.

In other words, with the right communication strategies aimed at structural change communities could place environmental health on the top of their priorities.

Conclusion

This chapter has presented different levels of strategies to address health communication for sustainable development. That concerns using participatory media to empower people to take health issues in their own hands and mobilize for social action. Empowerment means gaining more power to manage one's own assets, establishing social networks, and mobilizing social support. All this can be enhanced while using participatory media for social and structural change.

Group and structural levels of intervention are there to provide structures, resources, and opportunities for capacity building and networking. The media alone won't be able to change health behavior and the community direction. It is all about the people who use the media for the benefits of the community. Sustainability is a long-term perspective that requires commitment, perseverance, planning, policies, good governance and accountability.

References

Barker, M., Barker, D., Bormann, N. (2013). *Social Media Marketing. A Strategic Approach.* Australia: South-Western Cengage Learning.

Granich, R. & Mermin, J. (1999). *HIV Health & Your Community. A Guide for Action.* Standford, CA: Stanford University Press.

Hayes, B. M. & Aspray, W. (2010). The Informatics of Diabetes: A Research Agenda for the Socially and Institutionally Sensitive Use of Information Technology to Improve Healthcare. In B. M. Hayes & W. Aspray (Eds.) *Health Informatics. A Patient-Centered Approach to Diabetes.* Cambridge, MA & London: the MIT Press, pp. 3-81.

Jones, R. H. & Hafner, C. (2012). *Understanding Digital Literacies. A Practical Introduction.* London and New York: Routledge.

Li, W. et al. (2006). Animal Orignis of the Severe Acute Respiratory Syndrome Coronavirus: Insight from ACE2-S-Protein Interactions. *Journal of Virology.* May 80 (9), pp. 4211-4219 (Doi: 10.1128/JVI.80.9.4211-4219.2006) (http://jvi.asm.org/content/80/9/4211.full, accessed on Janurary 24th, 2016).

Mihailidis, P. (2015). Media Literacy and Mediated Communities: Emerging Perspectives for Digital Culture. In M. Shumow (Ed.) *Mediated Communities. Civic Voices, Empowerment and Media Literacy in the Digital Era*. New York: Peter Lang., pp.15-29.

Prasad, K. (2009 b). *Communication for Development. Reinventing Theory and Action. Volume 2. Advanced Development Communication*. Delhi: B. R. Publishing Corporation

UNAIDS & Penn State (1999). *Communication Framework for HIV/AIDS*. Geneva-University Park, PA: the Joint United Nations Programme on HIV/AIDS and the Pennsylvania State University.

World Health Organization Regional Office for Europe (2013). *A European Policy Framework and Strategy for the 21st Century*. Cohenhagen: World Health Organization (WHO) Regional Office for Europe.

Websites

PBS 2015 b
http://www.pbs.org/wgbh/pages/frontline/sickaroundtheworld/, accessed June 24, 2015.

Wellness city.co.th 2015
https://www.youtube.com/watch?v=poS-t_nYFrE, accessed on January 23rd, 2016.

Chapter 9

BY WAY OF CONCLUSION: EFFECTIVE HEALTH COMMUNICATION FOR SUSTAINABLE DEVELOPMENT

As explained throughout this book, old and newmedia have shaped the way people relate to one another on health related issues. The digital or social media, with their multi-modalities or mashups on multiple tools, have further accelerated these processes. For instance, Facebook offers photo albums, e-mail platforms, instant messaging programs, and blogs (Jones & Hafner 2012: 10). We have become self-mass communicators or part of mediated communities or interconnected networks. We can extend our communities beyond the physical boundaries through interconnectivity – connecting with other digital networks or the mass media. Recently, the mass media have merged with other types of media to form media convergences, such as vlogger or video blogger and internet radio, and we could link our network to larger networks for trustworthiness of information or for more professional investigations on certain types of news or information. We interact with one another both in real time or in a synchronous mode, and in delayed time or asynchronous mode, as we can save the messages and videos for later. Thanks to the multimodality of the digital media, we can chat via social media programs; we can video call people via our smart phones or laptops/tablets/ iPads; we can send instant messages, photos, opinions, or repost news or texts to others; or we can respond to news and opinions by commenting to the mass media messages online.

We all know by now that communication about/for health is not just sending health messages to stakeholders in a one-way fashion. Traditionally, two-way communication is recommended for feedback. However, with the current interconnectivity multiple ways of communication are on the rise. Digital communication has shaped our communication mode and culture by way of language use (such as acronyms e.g., LOL, creative use of punctuation, less attention to standard spelling, etc.); the way we use symbols (such as emoticons or digital stickers or keyboard generated graphics); the way we engage in daily life beyond the traditional phyical space, the way we identify our identities, the way we share our information, and the way we organize ourselves for the community interests or well-being (Jones & Hafner 2012: 66).

However, in addition to digital communication, we are still relying on news and information through the traditional mass media of television, radio, and newspapers. We still call each other on phones. We still visit places and people. We still try to personally meet each other to have a 'good time.'

Above all we need professional health communicators who can guide stakeholders in a community to avoid "health mythology" propagated by digital participatory tools, such as chat rooms, blogs, and posts on the social media networks, that may transmit information with limited factual data, wrong advice on disease prevention, or wrong health behaviors (Hayes & Aspray 2010: 27).

New ways of communication have strengthened our traditional ways of communication. That is a strategy a health communicator must keep in mind. Health communicators, as well as stakeholders, are expected to be digital media literates. To engage the interested public and stakeholders, health communicators need to access the digital culture of each age group. They must help young and old to understand their individual agency – how their digital voices (personal behaviors and words online) can contribute to dialogues in the digital public sphere; and their social agency—how they acknowledge those who are exposed to their digital voices, be it family, friends, peers, or acquaintances (Mihailidis 2015: 21). Moreover, all stakeholders in the community should be included—so that they have a sense of belonging to the community—and encouraged to sustain their direct engagement via mediated technologies, being both producers and consumers in the digital public sphere (Mihailidis 2015: 22-23). Sharing of information online can lead to engagement when the communities have a sense of value of joint dialogues; those common values, pushing towards actions, need mediated tools to join with other networks (Mihailidis 2015: 24-25).

Health communication strategies presented in this book are based on the understanding that there are many factors underpinning health. Starting from the paradigm or framework of addressing health at an individual, group, and structural level, we need to realize the impact of globalization and social determinants on health. Health literacy and media literacy are necessary for health communicators and stakeholders to communicate effectively about/on health. The knowledge of media technology, especially new media, and new developments in the Internet and on mobile devices need to be maintained for new strategies. However, we need to be aware of the importance of communication skills as well. Therefore, intercultural communication is essential to understand others and collaborate with others. Health communication is not a one-man-show process. It needs collaboration from all sectors in society. Sustainability in health can only be achieved once health equality is a reality.

Being a Thai national, I wish to close by reminding us of the strategies promoted by King Bhumibol or King Rama IX. Sustainability is what we gain from: (1) systematic fact gathering; (2) explore from the inside outward; (3) micro-focus on problem solving; (4) work step by step; (5) geosocial-based development; (6) think holistically or seeing the whole picture; (7) avoid textbook rigidity; (8) economize, emphasize simplicity to maximize benefit; (9) simplify complicated projects; (10) emphasize participation; (11) think of the common good; (12) have a one stop service for the people to save money and cost; (13) remember that nature is its own doctor; (14) don't fight evil with evil (in the case of nature that means, e.g., using natural weeds such as water hyacinth to absorb pollutants in water ways); (15) plant a forest in people's hearts (meaning train people the love for trees and nature); (16) our loss is our gain. Think about indirect ways that we gain from financial loss or sacrifice; (17) emphasize self-reliance; (18) create the ability to live comfortably and to eat decently; (19) emphasize a sufficient economy to control greed and excessive consumption; (20) build loyalty, honesty, and sincerity; (21) work happily; (22) have perseverance, be persistent and determined; and (23) know one another, love one another, and live in unity within your community.

REFERENCES

Hayes, B. M. & Aspray, W. (2010). The Informatics of Diabetes: A Research Agenda for the Socially and Institutionally Sensitive Use of Information Technology to Improve Health Care. In B. M. Hayes & W. Aspray (Eds.) *Health Informatics. A Patient-Centered Approach to Diabetes.* Cambridge, MA & London: the MIT Press, pp. 3-81.

Jones, R. H. & Hafner, C. (2012). *Understanding Digital Literacies. A Practical Introduction.* London and New York: Routledge.

Mihailidis, P. (2015). Media Literacy and Mediated Communities: Emerging Perspectives for Digital Culture. In M. Shumow (Ed.) *Mediated Communities. Civic Voices, Empowerment and Media Literacy in the Digital Era*. New York: Peter Lang., pp.15-29.

Bibliography

Agyeman, J. (2013). *Introducing Just Sustainabilities. Policy, Planning, and Practice*. London-New York: Zed Books.

Albrecht, T. L. & Adelmen, M. B. (1987). *Communicating Social Support*. Newbury Park, CA: Sage.

Albrecht, T. L. & Goldsmith, D. J. (2003). Social Support, Social Networks, and Health. In T. L. Thompson, A. Dorsey, K. I. Miller, R. Parrott (Eds.) *Handbook of Health Communication*. New York-London: Lawrence Erlbaum Associates., pp. 263-284.

Anderson, J. A. (1996). *Communication Theory. Epistemological Fou*ndations. New York-London: the Guilford Press.

Anderson, N. B. & Armstead, C. A. (1995). Toward Understanding the Association of Socio-economic Status and Health: A New Challenge for the Biophychosocial approach. *Psychosomatic Medicine* 57(1995): 213-225.

Anitei, S. (2007). Top 10 Infectious Diseases That Have Killed Millions of People. (http://news.softpedia.com/news/Top-10-Infectious-Diseases-That-Have-Killed-Most-People-70741.shtml, accessed on January 29th, 2016).

Babrow, A. S. & Mattson, M. (2003). Theorizing about Health Communication. In T. L. Thompson, A. Dorsey, K. I. Miller, and R. Parrot (Eds.) *Handbook of Health Communication*. New York-London: Lawrence Erlbaum Associates, Inc., pp. 35-61.

Baer, H. A., Singer, M. & Susser, I. (1997). *Medical Anthropology and the World System: A Critical Perspective*. Westport CT: Bergin & Garvey.

Barker, M., Barker, D., Bormann, N. & Neher, K. (2013). *Social Media Marketing. A Strategic Approach*. Australia: South-Western Cengage Learning.

Barrie, K. (2012). *Alcohol. Policy and Practice in Health and Social Care*. Edinburgh, Scotland: Dunedin Academic Press Ltd.

Baum, F., MacDougall, C., & Smith, D. (2006). Participatory Action Research. In *J Epidemiol Community Health*., 60: 854-857. (Doi: 10.1136/jech.2004.028662).

Bee, P. (2013). *The Food Swap Diet*. London: Piatkus.

Berger, P. L. & Luckmann, T. (1966). *The Social Construction of Reality: A Treatise in the Sociology of Knowledge*. New York: Doubleday & Co.

Berrigan, F. J. (1979). *Community Communications. The Role of Community Media in Development*. Paris: UNESCO.

Bird, C. E., Conrad, P., & Fremont, A. M. (2000). Medical Sociology at the Millennium. In C. E. Bird, P. Conrad, & A. M. Fremont (Eds.) *Handbook of Medical Sociology* (5th Ed.) Upper Saddle NJ: Prentice-Hall, Inc., pp. 1-10.

Blauner, R. (1972). *Racial Oppression in America*. New York: Harper.

Boyd-Barrett, O. (2015). *Media Imperialism*. Los Angeles-London-New Dehli-Singapore-Washington DC: SAGE Publications Inc.

Brewer, N. T. & Rimer, B. K. (2008). Perspectives on Health Behavior Theories that Focus on Individuals. In K. Glanz, B. K. Rimer & K. Viswanath (Eds.) *Health Behavior and Health Education. Theory, Research, and Practice*. (4th ed.) San Francisco, CA: Jossey-Bass, pp.149-165.

Brown, A. (1995). *Organisational Culture*. London: Pitman Publishing.

Brownell, A. & Shumaker, S. A. (1985). Where Do We Go from Here? The Policy Implications of Social Support. *Journal of Social Issues*, 41, 111-121.

Brundtland, G. H. & World Commission on Environment and Development. (1987). *Our Common Future* (vol. 383). Oxford: Oxford University Press.

Brunner, E. & Marmot, M. (1999). Social Organization Stress, and Health. In M. Marmot & R. G. Wilkinson (Eds.), *Social Determinants of Health*. Oxford, U.K: Oxford University Press, pp. 17-43.

Butterfoss, F. D., Kegler, M. C. & Francisco, V. T. (2008). Mobilizing Organizations for Health Promotion. Theories of Organizational Change In K. Glanz, B. K. Rimer & K. Viswanath (Eds.) *Health Behavior and Health Education. Theory, Research, and Practice*. (4th ed.) San Francisco, CA: Jossey-Bass, pp. 335-361.

Campbell, T. C. & Chen, J. (1994). Diet and Chronic Degenerative Diseases. A Summary of Results from an Ecology Study in Rural China. In N. J. Temple & D. P. Burkitt (Eds.) *Western Diseases. Their Dietary Prevention and Reversibility*. Totowa, NJ: Humana Press, pp. 67-118.

Cardello H. & Garr, D. (2010). *Stuffed. An Insider's Look at Who's (Really) Making America Fat and How the Food Industry Can Fix It*. New York: Ecco (an Imprint of Harper Collins Publishers).

Carey, J. W. (1992). *Communication as Culture: Essays on Media and Society*. New York-London: Routledge.

Carnegie, R., McKee, N., Dick, B., Reitemeier, P. et al. (2000). Making Change Possible: Creating and Enabling Environment. In N. McKee, E. Manoncourt, C. S. Yoon, and R. Carnegie (Eds.) *Involving People Evolving Behavior*. Penang: Southbound, pp.157-211.

Carnegie, R. & Weisen, R. B. (2000). The Ability to Act: Strengthening People's Life Skills. In N. McKee, E. Manoncourt, C. S. Yoon, and R. Carnegie (Eds.) *Involving People Evolving Behavior*. Penang: Southbound, pp.121-154.

Castells, M. (2013). *Communication Power*. Oxford, U.K: Oxford University Press.

Champion, V. L. & Skinner, C. S. (2008). The Health Belief Model. In K. Glanz, B. K. Rimer & K. Viswanath (Eds.) *Health Behavior and Health Education. Theory, Research, and Practice*. (4th ed.) San Francisco, CA: Jossey-Bass, pp. 45-65.

Chan, M. (2013). Foreword. In *Health 2020. A European Policy Framework and Strategy for the 21st Century*. Copenhagen: World Health Organization (WHO) Regional Office for Europe, p. 8.

Chen, G.-M. & Starosta, W. J. (2004). “Communication among Cultural Diversities.” In G.M. Chen & W. J. Starosta (Eds.) *Dialogue among Diversities*. Washington D.C: National Communication Association, pp. 3-15.

Cohen, D. (2006). *Globalization and Its Enemies* (J. B. Baker, Trans.) Cambridge, MA: Massachusetts Institute of Technology Press.

Cordell, D. D., Gregory, J. W., & Piche, V. (1992). The Demographic Reproduction of Health and Disease: Colonial Centeral African Republic and Contemporary Burkina Faso. In S. Feierman & J. M. Janzen (Eds.) *The Social Basis of Health and Healing in Africa.* Berkeley: University of California Press.

Cox, R. & Pezzullo, P. (2016). *Environmental Communication and the Public Sphere* (4th ed.) Los Angelis-London-New Dehli-Singapore-Washington DC-Boston: Sage.

Davis-Case, D. (1989). *Community Forestry. Participatory Assessment, Monitoring and Evaluation*. Rome: Food and Agriculture Organization of the United Nations.

De Graaf, J., Wann, D. & Naylor, T. H. (2014). *Affluenza: How Overconsumption is Killing Us—and How We Can Fight Back (3rd ed.)* San Francisco: Berrett-Koehler Publishers, Inc.

De Rivero, O. (2001). *The Myth of Development*. London and New York: Zed Books.

Dolinoy, D. C. (2015). Early-Life Exposures and the Epigenome: Interactions between Nutrients and the Environment. In E. Ho & F. Domann (Eds.) *Nutrition and Epigenetics*, pp. 3-52.

Du Pre, A. (2014). Communicating about Health. (4th ed.) New York-Oxford: Oxford University Press.

Duhigg, C. (2013). *The Power of Habit. Why We Do What We Do and How to Change.* London: Random House Books.

Dutta, M. & Zoller, H. (2008). Theoretical Foundations. Interpretive, Critical, and Cultural Approaches to Health Communication. In H. M. Zoller & M. J. Dutta (Eds.) *Emerging Perspectives in Health Communication. Meaning, Culture, and Power*. New York and London: Routledge, pp. 1-27.

Dutta, M. J. (2008). *Communicating Health*. Malden MA: Polity Press.

Dyll-Myklebust, L. & Zwane, D. (2015). Uncovering Barriers to Bilharzia Prevention Communication in Ugu District, South Africa: Lessons Learned Through Participatory Communication. *Communicare. Journal for Communication Sciences in Southern Africa*, pp. 65-81.

Egger, G. & Dixon, J. (2011). Non-nutrient Causes of Low-grade, Systemic inflammation: Support for a ‘Canary in the Mineshaft’ View of Obesity in Chronic Disease. *Obes Rev*, 12(5), pp. 339-345.

Elias, N. (1978). *What is Sociology?* London: Hutchinson.

Evans, D. (2006). How Social Marketing Works in Healthcare. *British Medical Journal*. May 20. 332(7551) pp. 1207-1210. (Doi: 10.1136/bmj.332.7551.1207-a).

Fairburn, C. G. (2008). *Cognitive Behavior Therapy and Eating Disorders*. New York: Guilford Press. (http://www.wales.nhs.uk/sitesplus/866/opendoc/225354, accessed on September 8th, 2015).

Fairclough, N. (1992). *Critical Language Awareness*. New York: Longman.

Farley, H. M. & Smith, Z. A. (2014). *Sustainability. If It’s Everything, Is It Nothing?* London-New York: Routledge.

Featherstone, M. (1996). Localism, Globalism, and Cultural Identity. In R. Wilson & W.

Dissanayake (Eds.) *Global Local: Cultural Productions and the Transnational Imaginary* Durham and London: Duke University Press., pp. 46-77.

Foucault, M. (1973). *The Birth of the Clinic*. London: Tavistock.

Fox, E. (2012). Rethinking Health Communication in Aid and Development. In R. Obregon & S. Waisbord (Eds.) *The Handbook of Global Health Communication*. West Sussex: Wiley-Blackwell, a John Wiley & Sons, Ltd., Publication, pp. 52-69.

Freire, P. (1993). *Education for Critical Consciousness*. New York: Continuum.

Fuchs, C. & Sandoval, M. (2015). The Political Economy of Capitalist and Alternative Social Media. In C. Atton (Ed.) *The Routledge Companion to Alternative and Community Media*. London-New York: Routledge.

Galanti, G. (2008). *Caring for Patients from Different Cultures* (4th ed.) Philadelphia: University of Pennsylvania Press.

Gannon, M. J. (2008). *Paradoxes of Culture and Globalization*. Los Angeles-London-New Delhi-Singapore: Sage Publications.

Geertz, C. (1983). *Local Knowledge*. New York: Basic Books, Inc.

Geertz, C. (1995). *After the Fact: Two Countries, four decades, one anthropologist*. Cambridge, MA: Harvard University Press.

Giddens, A. & Sutton, P. W. (2012). Chapter Summary for Chapter 9 The Life Course. (www.polity.co.uk/giddens7/studentresource/summaries/Student_summary_09.asp, accessed on June 3rd, 2015).

Giddens, A. (1990). *The Consequence of Modernity*. Cambridge: Polity Press.

Giddens, A., Duneier, M., Appelbaum, R. P., & Carr, D. (2014). *Introduction to Sociology*. New York-London: W. W. Norton & Company, Inc.

Gielen, A. C., McDonald, E. M., Gary, T. L. & Bone, L. R. (2008). Using the PRECEDE-PROCEED Model to Apply Health Behavior Theories. In K. Glanz, B. K. Rimer & K. Viswanath (Eds.) *Health Behavior and Health Education. Theory, Research, and Practice*. (4th ed.) San Francisco, CA: Jossey-Bass, pp. 407-433.

Gilbert, D. & Kahl, J. (1982). *The American Class Structure: A New Synthesis*. Homewood, IL: Dorsey.

Gilbert, D. (2008). *The American Class Structure in an Age of Growing Inequality*. (7th ed). Thousand Oaks, CA: Pine Forge.

Glanz, K. (2008). Improving Health Through Community Organization and Community Building. In K. Glanz, B. K. Rimer & K. Viswanath (Eds.) *Health Behavior and Health Education. Theory, Research, and Practice*. (4th ed.) San Francisco, CA: Jossey-Bass, pp.287-312.

Goldberg, R. (2014). *Understanding Contemporary Social Problems through Media*. Boulder-London: Paradigm Publishers.

Granich, R. & Mermin, J. (1999). *HIV Health & Your Community. A Guide for Action*. Standford, CA: Stanford University Press.

Green, L.W., Kreuter, M. W., Deeds, S. G., and Partridge, K. B. (1980*). Health Education Planning: A Diagnostic Approach*. Mountain View, CA: Mayfield.

Hackett, R. A. & Gurleyen, P. (2015). Beyond the Binaries? Alternative Media and Objective Journalism. In C. Atton (Ed.) *The Routledge Companion to Alternative and Community Media*. London-New York: Routledge.

Hall, E. T. (1959). *The Silent Language*. New York: Doubleday.

Hamilton, C. & Denniss, R. (2005). *Affluenza. When too Much is Never Enough*. Crows Nest NSW: Allen & Unwin.

Harris, R. L. & Seid, M. J. (2004). Globalization and Health in the New Millennium. In R. L. Harris & M. Seid (Eds.) *Globalization and Health*. Leiden & Boston: Brill, pp. 1-46.

Harris, S. (2010). *The Moral Landscape. How Science Can Determine Human Values*. New York-London-Toronto-Sydney: Free Press.

Hayes, B. M. & Aspray, W. (2010). The Informatics of Diabetes: A Research Agenda for the Socially and Institutionally Sensitive Use of Information Technology to Improve Health Care. In B. M. Hayes & W. Aspray (Eds.) *Health Informatics. A Patient-Centered Approach to Diabetes*. Cambridge, MA & London: the MIT Press, pp. 3-81.

Heaney, C. A. & Israel, B. A. (2008). Social Networks and Social Support. In K. Glanz, B. K. Rimer & K. Viswanath (Eds.) *Health Behavior and Health Education. Theory, Research, and Practice*. (4th ed.) San Francisco, CA: Jossey-Bass, pp.189-210.

Heinonen, A. & Domingo, D. (2008). Webblogs and Journalism: A Typology to Explore the Blurring Boundaries. *Nordicom Review*, 29(1), 3-15.

Held, D. & McGrew, A. (2007). *Globalization/Anti-globalization*. Cambridge-Malden MA: Polity Press.

Hepburn, S. J. (1988). Western Minds, Foreign Bodies. *Medical Anthropology Quarterly* 2, pp. 59-74.

Hepp, A. (2013). *Cultures of Mediatization*. (K. Tribe Trans.) Cambridge: Polity Press.

Heusca, R. (2008). Tracing the History of Participatory Communication Approaches to Development: A Critical Appraisal. In (J. Servaes ed.)*Communication for Development and Social Change*. Los Angeles: Sage.

HIV/AIDS Electronic Library. (2015). http://library.unesco-iicba.org/English/HIV_AIDS/cdrom%20materials/Poverty.htm, accessed on June 22nd, 2015.

Hjarvard, S. (2013). *The Mediatization of Culture and Society*. Routledge: London and New York.

Hofstede, G. (2001). *Culture's Consequences: Comparing Values, Behaviours, Institutions and Organizations across Nations* (2nd ed). Beverly Hills, CA: Sage Publications, Inc. (https://ad34c3acb3d2700a49a406cdff75053dd1fd8d65.googledrive.com/host/0B7aKRMPHsA89MmJrLTlRcFNSZG8/Seen%20in%20Their%20True%20Light%20(2012-05).pdf, accessed on June 26th, 2015).

Holm, N. (1997). An Integrated Role Theory for the Psychology of Religion: Concepts and Perspectives. In B. Spilka & D. McIntosh (Eds.) *The Psychology of Religion* Oxford: Westview Press., pp. 73-94. (http://search.ebscohost.com/login.aspx?direct=true&db=aph&AN=20921322&site=ehost-live)

Holmberg, C. B. (1998). *Sexualities and Popular Culture*. Sage Publications: Thousand Oaks.

Hong, E. (2000). *Globalization and the Impact on Health. A Third World View*. Document prepared for the People's Health Assembly, December 4-8, Savar, Bangladesh.

Hopkins, A. G. (2002). Introduction: Globalization – An Agenda for Historians. In A. G. Hopkins (Ed.), *Globalization in World History* (pp. 1-10). London: Pimlico.

Hopper, P. (2006). *Living with Globalization* Oxford. New York: Berg. (http://search.ebscohost.com/login.aspx?direct=true&db=aph&AN=20921322&site=ehost-live, accessed on June 8th, 2015).

Huang, Y. (2013). *Governing Health in Contemporary China*. New York: Routledge.

Hugman, R. & Bartolomei, L. (2014). The Ethics of Participation in Community Work Practice. In A. K. Larsen, V. Sewpaul & G. O. Hole (Eds.) *Participation in Community Work. International Perspectives*. London and New York: Routledge, pp. 19-29.

Human Development Report (2010). *The Real Wealth of Nations*. New York: United Nations Development Program. http: hdr.undp.org/en/media/HDR_2010_EN_Complete_reprint.pdf (accessed on June 21st, 2013)

Hung, L. S., (2003). The SARS Epidemic in Hong Kong: What Lessons Have We Learned? *Journal of the Royal Society of Medicine*. 96(8); 2003 August, (http://www.ncbi.nlm.nih.gov/pmc/articles/PMC539564/, accessed on Jan 12th, 2015).

Hunter, J., Marshall, J., Corcoran, K. and Leeder, S. (2013). A Positive Concept of Health—Interviews with Patients and Practitioners in an Integrative Medicine Clinic. *Complementary Therapies in Clinical Practice* 19, 197-203. http://dx.doi.org/10.1016/j.ctcp.2013.07.001, accessed on March 20th, 2015.

Irwin, H. (1989). Health Communication: The research agenda. *Media Information Australia*. 54, pp. 32-40.

Janzen, J.M. (2002). *The Social Fabric of Health: An Introduction to Medical Anthropology*. Boston: McGrawHill.

Jayasaro Bhikku (2012). *Seen in their true light*. Bangkok: Panyaprateep Foundation (www.panyaprateep.org).

Jones, R. H. & Hafner, C. (2012). *Understanding Digital Literacies. A Practical Introduction*. London and New York: Routledge.

Jun, J. & Worth, H. (2010). An Overview of China's HIV Epidemic. In J.Jun & H. Worth (Eds.) *HIV in China: Understanding the Social Aspects of the Epidemic*. Sydney: UNSW Press, pp. 13-41.

Kakar, V. N. (1987). *Communication in India's Family Planning—India's Experience*. New Delhi: National Institute of Health and Family Welfare.

Kandel, D. B., Wu, P., & Davies, M. (1994). Maternal smoking during pregnancy and smoking by adolescent daughters. *American Journal of Public Health*, 84, 1407-1413.

Kar, S. B., Alcalay, R. & Alex, S. (2001). The Evolution of Health Communication in the United States. In S.B.Kar, R. Alcalay & S. Alex (Eds.) *Health Communication. A Multicultural Perspective*. Thousand Oaks-London-New Delhi: Sage Publications, Inc., pp. 45-78.

Karl, M. (1999). Networks and Networking: Conclusions and Challenges. I. 1 Introduction. In M. Karl, A. Anand, F. Blankenberg, A. van den Ham, et al. (Eds.) *Measuring the Immeasurable. Planning Monitoring and Evaluation of Networks*. New Delhi: Women's Feature Service., pp. 17-26.

Karl, M. (1999). Networks and Networking: Conclusions and Challenges. In (M. Karl, A. Anand, F. Blankenberg, A. van den Ham, et al. eds.) *Measuring the Immeasurable. Planning Monitoring and Evaluation of Networks*. New Delhi: Women's Feature Service.

Kawachi, I. & Kennedy, B. P. (1997). Health and Social Cohesion: Why Care about Income Inequality? *British Medical Journal*, 314, pp. 1037-1040.

Kennedy, B., Kawachi, I., & Prothrow-Stith, D. (1996). Income Distribution and Mortality: Test of the Robin Hood Index in the United States. *British Medical Journal*, 312, pp. 1004-1007.

Kennedy, T. (2008). *Where the Rivers Meet the Sky. A Collaborative Approach to Participatory Development*. Penang: Southbound.

Kim, Y. M. (2012). *Critical Intercultural Communication Strategies in the Age of Glocalism*. Korea: Han Gukmoonhwasa.

Kivits, J. (2013). E-health and Renewed Sociological Approaches to Health and Illness. In K. Orton-Johnson & N. Prior (Eds.) *Digital Sociology. Critical Perspectives*. New York: Palgrave Macmillan., pp.213-226.

Kreps, G. L., & Thornton, B. C. (1992). *Health Communication: Theory & practice* (2nd ed.). Prospect Heights, IL: Waveland Press.

Lederman, L.C. (2010). Health Communication. The First Twenty-five Years. In J.W.Chesebro (Ed.) *A Century of Transformation. Studies in Honor of the 100th Anniversary of the Eastern Communication Association* (4th ed.), New York: Oxford University Press., pp. 236-254.

Lee, K. & Zwi, A. (2003). A Global Political Economy Approach to AIDS: Ideology, Interests and Implications. In K. Lee (Ed.) *Health Impacts of Globalization. Towards Global Governance*. Hampshire-New York: Palgrave Macmillan.

Lee, K. (2003). *Globalization and Health. An Introduction*. New York: Palgrave Macmillan.

Lee, K. (2004). Globalisation: What is it and how does it affect health? *The Medical Journal of Australia*, 180 (4), pp. 156-158. (https://www.mja.com.au/journal/2004/180/4/globalisation-what-it-and-how-does-it-affect-health, accessed on July 19th, 2015).

Lee, K. (2005). Global Social Change and Health. In K. Lee & J. Collin (Eds.) *Global Change and Health*. New York: Open University Press/ McGraw-Hill Education, pp. 13-27.

Lerner, D. (1958). *The Passing of Traditional Society: Modernizing the Middle East*. New York: Free Press.

Levy, B. S. & Sidel, V. W. (2006). The Nature of Social Injustice and Its Impact on Public Health. In B. S. Levy & V. W. Sidel (Eds.), *Social Injustice and Public Health*. Oxford-New York: Oxford University Press., pp. 5-21.

Li, W. et al. (2006). Animal Orignis of the Severe Acute Respiratory Syndrome Coronavirus: Insight from ACE2-S-Protein Interactions. *Journal of Virology*. May 80 (9), pp. 4211-4219 (Doi: 10.1128/JVI.80.9.4211-4219.2006) (http://jvi.asm.org/content/80/9/4211.full, accessed on Janurary 24th, 2016).

Lie, R. & Servaes, J. (2015). Disciplines in the Field of Communication for Development and Social Change. *Communication Theory*. 25(2015), pp. 244-258.

Lie, R. (2003). *Spaces of Intercultural Communication: An Interdisciplinary Introduction to Communication, Culture, and Globalizing/Localizing Identities*. New Jersey: Hampton Press, Inc.

Linker, M. (2015). *Intellectual Empathy. Critical Thinking for Social Justice*. University of Michigan Press: Ann Arbor.

Louw, E. (2005). *The Media and Political Process*. London-Thousand Oaks-New Dehli: Sage Publications.

Lupton, D. (1994). Toward the Development of Critical Health Communication Praxis. *Health Communication*. 6(1), pp. 55-67.

MacBride, S. (1980). *Many voices, one world. Communication and society. Today and tomorrow* (S. MacBride Ed.) Paris: UNESCO.

MacLachlan, M. (1997). *Culture and Health*. New York: John Wiley & Sons.

Madden, T. J., Ellen, P. S., & Ajzen, I. (1992). A Comparison of the Theory of Planned Behavior and the Theory of Reasoned Action. *Personality and Social Psychology Bulletin*. Feb. 1992 18: 3-9.

Malikhao, P. (2007). *HIV/AIDS Prevention Strategies in Two Thai Communities: Buddhist and Christian*. Ph.D. thesis. Brisbane: University of Queensland.

Malikhao, P. (2012). *Sex in the Village. Culture, Religion and HIV/AIDS in Thailand.* Southbound & Silkworm Publishers: Penang-Chiang Mai, 238pp. (ISBN: 978-983-9054-55-2).

Malikhao, P. (2013 a). Communication for Development and Sustainability. *Media Development*, 3, pp. 1-5.

Malikhao, P. (2013 b). Understanding the Spread of HIV/AIDS in Thailand. In J. Servaes (Ed.), *Sustainability, Participation and Culture in Communication*. Intellect/University of Chicago Press: Bristol/Chicago, pp.273-292.

Manyozo, L. (2012). Community Media, Health Communication, and Engagement. A Theoretical Matrix. In R. Obregon & S. Waisbord (Eds.) *The Handbook of Global Health Communication*. West Sussex: Wiley-Blackwell, pp. 233-250.

Marchlewicz, E. H., Anderson, O. S., & Dolinoy, D.C. (2015). Early-Life Exposures and the Epigenome. Interactions between Nutrients and the Environment. In E. Ho & F. Domann (Eds.) *Nutrition and Epigenetics*. London-New York: CRC Press, pp. 3-52.

Marmot, M. & Bell, R. (2006). The Socioeconomically Disadvantage. In B. S. Levy & V. W. Side (Ed.) *Social Injustice and Public Health*. Oxford-New York: Oxford University Press.

Martin, J. N. & Nakayama, T. K. (2004). *Intercultural Communication in Contexts*. McGraw Hill: Boston.

Martin, J. N. & Nakayama, T. K. (2010). *Intercultural Communication in Contexts* (5th ed.) New York: McGraw-Hill.

Martin, J. N. & Nakayama, T. K. (2014). *Experiencing Intercultural Communication. An Introduction*. New York: McGraw-Hill.

McElroy, A. & Townsend, P. (1979). *Medical Anthropology in Ecological Perspective*. North Scituate, MA: Duxbury Press.

McKee, N., Manoncourt, E., Yoon, C. S., & Carnegie, R. (2000*). Involving People. Evolving Behavior*. Penang: Southbound.

McQuail, D. & Windahl, S. (1993). *Communication Models for the Study of Mass Communication*. London and New York: Longman.

McQuail, D. (2005). *McQuail's Mass Communication Theory* (5th ed.) London-Thousand Oaks-New Delhi: Sage Publications.

Melkote, S. R. & Steeves, H.L. (2001). Communication Approach in the Modernizing of the Third World. In *Communication for Development in the Third World*. (2^{nd}ed.). New Delhi-Thousand Oaks-London: Sage Publications,pp.103-147.

Mihailidis, P. (2015). Media Literacy and Mediated Communities: Emerging Perspectives for Digital Culture. In M. Shumow (Ed.) *Mediated Communities. Civic Voices, Empowerment and Media Literacy in the Digital Era*. New York: Peter Lang., pp.15-29.

Mirowsky, J., Ross, C. & Reynolds, J. (2000). Link between Social Status and Health Status. In C. E. Bird, P. Conrad & A. M. Fremont (Eds.) *Handbook of Medical Sociology*. Upper Saddle River, N.J: Prentice-Hall, Inc., pp. 68-78.

Mohammed, S. N. (2011). *Communication and the Globalization of Culture*. Lanham-Boulder-New York-Toronto-Plymouth, UK: Lexington Books.

Montano, D. E. & Kasprzyk, D. (2008). Theory of Reasoned Action, Theory of Planned Behavior, and the Integrated Behavioral Model. In K. Glanz, B. K. Rimer & K. Viswanath (Eds.) *Health Behavior and Health Education. Theory, Research, and Practice*. (4th ed.) San Francisco, CA: Jossey-Bass, pp. 67-96.

Moore, M., Gould, P. & Keary, B. (2003). Global Urbanization and Impact on Health. *International Journal of Hygiene and Environmental Health*, 206, pp. 269-278.

Morrison, V. & Bennett, P. (2006). *Introduction to Health Psychology*. Harlow, Essex, England; New York: Pearson/Prentice Hall.

Nash, K. (2000). *Contemporary Political Sociology*. London: Blackwell Publishers.

Nestle, M. (2006). *What to Eat*. New York: North Point Press.

Nestle, M. (2007). *Food Politics. How the Food Industry Influences Nutrition and Health*. Berkeley-Los Angeles-London: University of California Press.

Nestle, M. (2009). *What to Eat*. New York: North Point Press.

Nestle, M. (2013). *Food Politics. How the Food Industry Influences Nutrition and Health*. Berkeley-Los Angeles-London: University of California Press.

Nestle, M. (2013). *Food Politics. How the Food Industry Influences Nutrition and Health* (10th ed.). Berkeley-Los Angeles-London: University of California Press.

Neuman, W. R. (1991). *The Future of the Mass Audience*. Cambridge, U.K: Cambridge University Press.

Nisbett, R. E. (2003). *The Geography of Thought: How Asians and Westerners Think Differently and Why*. New York-London-Toronto-Sydney-Singapore: The Free Press.

Oldenburg, B. & Glanz, K. (2008). Diffusion of Innovations. Montano, D. E. & Kasprzyk, D. (2008). Theory of Reasoned Action, Theory of Planned Behavior, and the Integrated Behavioral Model. In K. Glanz, B. K. Rimer & K. Viswanath (Eds.) *Health Behavior and Health Education. Theory, Research, and Practice*. (4th ed.) San Francisco, CA: Jossey-Bass, pp. 313-333.

Omoto, A. (2005). *Processes of Community Change and Social Action*. Mahwah: Lawrence Erlbaum Associates.

Pajnik, M. (2015). Changing Citizenship, Practising (Alternative) Politics. In C. Atton (Ed.) *The Routledge Companion to Alternative and Community Media*. London and New York: Routledge, pp. 113-122.

PANOS (2006). *Speaking Freely, Being Strong: HIV Social Movements, Communication and Inclusive Social Change*. London: The Panos Institute.

Papa, M., Singhal, A., & Papa, W. (2006). *Organizing for Social Change. A Dialectic Journey of Theory and Praxis*. New Delhi: Sage.

Parrot, R. (2009). *Talking about Health. Why Communication Matters*. Malden, M.A: Wiley-Blackwell.

Parrott, A. C. (1999). Does cigarette smoking cause stress? *American Psychologist*, 54, 817-820.

Paul-Edwards, J. (2013). What might Web 4.0 Look Like and Should You be Preparing? IMedia Connection website (http://www.imediaconnection.com/content/34206.asp, accessed on November 2nd, 2015).

Payutto, P. A. (1998). *Sustainable Development* (3rd ed.). Bangkok: Buddhatham Foundation.

Payutto, P. A. (2003). *Sustainable Development* (6th ed.). Bangkok: Komol Keemthong Foundation Press.

Payutto, P.A. (2006). *Sukhapava Ong Ruam Naew Buddha (Holistic well-being the Buddhist Way).* (http://www.fungdham.com/download/book/payutto/490109-sukhapava.pdf).

Payutto, P.A. (2007). *A Buddhist Solution for the Twenty-first Century* (17th ed.) Bangkok: Pimsuay Printing.

Payutto, P.A. (2013). *Sustainable Development* (13th ed.) Bangkok: Komol Keemthong Foundation.

Perls, T. T. & Fretts, R. C. (1988). Why Women Live Longer than Men. *Scientific American*, pp. 100-103.

Perrings, C. (2014). *Our Uncommon Heritage. Biodiversity Change, Ecosysem Services, and Human Well-being*. Cambridge: Cambridge University Press.

Pollard, T. M. (2008). *Western Diseases. An Evolutionary Perspective*. Cambridge: Cambridge University Press.

Powell, J. L. & Steel, R. (2011). Revisiting Appadurai: Globalizing Scapes in a Globalized World-The Pervasiveness of Economic and Cultural Power. *International Journal of Innovative Interdisciplinary Research 1*, December 1: 74-80.

Prasad, K. (2009 a). *Communication for Development. Reinventing Theory and Action. Volume 1. Understanding Communication*. Delhi: B.R. Publishing Corporation.

Prasad, K. (2009 b). *Communication for Development. Reinventing Theory and Action. Volume 2. Advanced Development Communication*. Delhi: B. R. Publishing Corporation.

Prochaska, J. O., Redding, C. A., & Evers, K. E. (2008). The Transtheoretical Model and Stages of Change. In K. Glanz, B. K. Rimer & K. Viswanath (Eds.) *Health Behavior and Health Education. Theory, Research, and Practice*. (4th ed.) San Francisco, CA: Jossey-Bass, pp. 97-121.

Rieker, P. P. & Bird, C. E. (2000). Sociological Explanations of Gender Differences in Mental and Physical Health. In C. E. Bird, P. Conrad, & A. M. Fremont (Eds.) *Handbook of Medical Sociology* (5th Ed.) Upper Saddle NJ: Prentice-Hall, Inc., pp. 98-113.

Robert, S. A. & House, J. S. (2000). Socioeconomic Inequalities in Health: An Enduring Sociological Problem. In C. E. Bird, P. Conrad, & A. M. Fremont (Eds.) *Handbook of Medical Sociology* (5th Ed.) Upper Saddle NJ: Prentice-Hall, Inc., pp.79-111.

Robertson, R. (1972). *The Sociological Interpretation of Religion*. Oxford: Basil Blackwell.

Rostow, W. W. (1953). *The Process of Economic Growth*. Oxford: Clarendon Press.

Ruiz-Nunez, B., Pruimboom, L., Dijck-Brouwer, D.A. J., Muskiet, F. A. J. (2013). Lifestyle and Nutritional Imbalances Associated with Western Diseases: Causes and Consequences of Chronic Systemic Low Grade Inflammation in an Evolutionary Context. *The Journal of Nutritional Biochemistry* 24(7), pp. 1183-1201. (doi: 10.1016/j/jnutbio.2013.02.009).

Ryan, R. M. & Deci, E. L. (2002). Overview of Self-Determination Theory: An Oganismic Dialectical Perspective. In E. L. Deci & R. M. Ryan (Eds.) *Handbook of Self-Determination Research*. Rochester, NY: the University of Rochester Press, pp.3-33.

Sachs,W. (2013). Liberating the World from Development. *New Internationalist*. 460, March, p. 25.

Sallis, J. F., Owen, N. & Fisher, E. B. (2008). Ecological Models of Health Behavior. In K. Glanz, B.K. Rimer, K Viswanath (Eds.) *Health Behavior and Health Education. Theory, Research, and Practice*. (4th ed.). San Francisco: John Wiley & Sons, Inc., pp. 465-485.

Sarafino, E. P. (2006). *Health Psychology. Biopsychosocial Interactions*. (5th ed.) N.J: John Wiley & Sons, Inc.

Schafer, R. (1968). *Aspects of internalization*. New York: International Universities Press.

Schiavo, R. (2007). What is Health Communication?. In *Health Communication. From Theory to Practice*. San Francisco: Jossey-Bass, pp. 3-29.

Schneider, M. (2006). *Introduction to Public Health*. Boston: Jones and Bartlett Publishers.

Scholte, J. A. (2005). *Globalization: A Critical Introduction*. Basingstoke: Palgrave Macmillan.

Seidman, C., Silberg, W. M., and Patrick, K. (2013). Contemporary Issues in Scientific Communication and Public Health Education. In J.W. Holsinger Jr. (Ed.) *Contemporary Public Health*. Kentucky: the University Press of Kentucky, pp. 171-191.

Sernau, S. (2014). *Social Inequality in a Global Age* (4th ed.) Los Angeles-London-New Delhi-Singapore-Washington DC: Sage.

Servaes, J. & Lie, R. (2014). New Challenges for Communication for Sustainable Development and Social Change: a Review Essay. *Journal of Multicultural Discourses*. (http://dx.doi.org/10.1080/17447143.2014982655).

Servaes, J. & Malikhao, P. (2008). Development Communication Approaches in an International Perspective. In J. Servaes (Ed.) *Communication for Development and Social Change*. Los Angeles: Sage, pp. 158-179.

Servaes, J. & Malikhao, P. (2009). Advocacy Strategies for Health Communication. *Public Relations Review*. Doi: 10.1016/j. pubrev.2009.08.017.

Servaes, J. & Malikhao, P. (2010). Advocacy Strategies for Health Communication. *Public Relations Review*, pp. 42-49. (Doi: 10.1016/j.pubrev.2009.08.017).

Servaes, J. (1999). *Communication for Development: One World, Multiple Cultures* (1st ed.) Cresskill, New Jersey: Hampton Press, Inc.

Servaes, J. (2007). Harnessing the UN System into a Common Approach on Communication for Development. *The International Communication Gazette*, Sage, 69, 6, pp. 483-507. (http://gaz.sagepub.com).

Servaes, J. (2013). Introduction: Imperatives for a Sustainable Future. In J. Servaes (Ed.) *Sustainable Development and Green Communication. African and Asian Perspectives*. New York: Palgrave Macmillan, pp. 1-39.

Servaes, J., Polk, E., Shi, S., Reilly, D. & Yukupitijage, T. (2012). Towards a Framework of Sustainability Indicators for 'Communication for Development and Social Change' Projects. *The International Communication Gazette*, pp. 1-25. (Doi: 10.1177/1748048511432598).

Servaes, J., Polk, E., Shi, S., Reilly, D., et.al (2012). Sustainability Testing for Development Projects. *Development in Practice*. 22 (1).

Share, J. (2015). *Media Literacy is Elementary. Teaching Youth to Critically Read and Create Media* (2nd ed.). New York: Peter Lang.

Sheron, B. K. & Deborah, V. (1997). *Crosstalk: Communicating in a Multicultural Workplace*. Upper Saddle River, NJ: Prentice Hall.

Silverblatt, A., Smith, A., Miller, D., Smith, J. et al. (2014). *Media Literacy. Keys to Interpreting Media Messages* (4th ed.). Santa Barbara, CA: Praeger.

Singhal, A. & Rogers, E. M. (1999). *Entertainment-education: a communication strategy for social change*. Mahwah, NJ: Lawrence Erlbaum Associates.

Smith, J. C. & Medalia, C. (2015). Health Insurance Coverage in the United States: 2014.

Current Population Reports. September. (https://www.census.gov/content/dam/Census/library/publications/2015/demo/p60-253.pdf, accessed on February 22, 2016).

Sorensen, K., Van den Broucke, S., Fullam, J., Doyle, G., Pelikan, J., et al. (2012). Health Literacy and Public Health: A Systematic Review and Integration of Definitions and Models. *BMC Public Health* 12:80. (http://www.biomedcentral.com/1471-2458/12/80).

Spector, R. E. (2000). *Cultural Diversity in Health & Illness.* (5th ed.) Upper Saddle, N.J: Prentice Hall Health.

Storey, J. D., Saffitz, G. B., Rimon, J. G. (2008). Social Marketing. In K. Glanz, B. K. Rimer & K. Viswanath (Eds.) *Health Behavior and Health Education. Theory, Research, and Practice.* (4th ed.) San Francisco, CA: Jossey-Bass, pp. 435-464.

Suggs, L. S. & Ratzan, S. C. (2012). Global E-health Communication. In R. Obregon & S. Waisbord (Eds.) *The Handbook of Global Health Communication.* West Sussex: Wiley-Blackwell, pp. 251-273.

Summerfield, L. M. (2012). *Nutrition, Exercise, & Behavior. An Integrated Approach to Weight Management.* Belmont, CA: Wadsworth.

Sztompka, P. (1993). *The Sociology of Social Change.* Cambridge, U.S.A.: Basil.

The Levin Institute-The State University of New York (2014). Globalization 101. (http://www.globalization101.org/diseases-go-global/, accessed on Jan 11th, 2015).

Thompson, J. (1995). *The Media and Modernity. A Social Theory of the Media.* Cambridge: Polity Press.

Thompson, T. L., Dorsey, A., Miller, K. I., & Parrott, R. (2003). *Handbook of Health Communication.* (T. L. Thompson, A. Dorsey, K. I. Miller & R. Parrott Eds.) New York-London: Lawrence Erlbaum Associates.

Trochim, W. M. K. (2006). Positivism & Post-Postitivism. (http://www.socialresearch methods.net/kb/positvsm.php, accessed on April 7th, 2015).

Turner, J. W. (2003). Telemedicine: Expanding Health Care into Virtual Environments. In T. L. Thompson, A. Dorsey, K. I. Miller & R. Parrott (Eds.) *Handbook of Health Communication.* New York-London: Lawrence Erlbaum Associates, pp. 515-535.

Turow, J. (2014). *Media Today. Mass Communication in a Converging World* (5th ed.) New York: Routledge.

UNAIDS & Penn State (1999). *Communication Framework for HIV/AIDS.* Geneva-University Park, PA: the Joint United Nations Programme on HIV/AIDS and the Pennsylvania State University.

UNESCO (2007). *Harnessing Communication to Achieve the Millennium Development Goals.* Paris: UNESCO.

United Nations (2008). *Achieving Sustainable Development and Promoting Development Cooperation.* New York: United Nations.

US Department of Health and Human Services (HSS) (2000). *Healthy people 2010: Understanding and Improving Health.* Washington, DC: US Government Printing Office.

Uzelac, A. (2008). How to Understand Digital Culture: Digital Culture—a Resource for a Knowledge Society? In A. Uzelac & B. Cvjeticanin (Eds.) *Digital Culture: The - Changing Dynamics. Zagreb, Croatia*: Institute for International Relations., pp. 7-21.

Verma, S. (2011). *International Media Communication in a Global Age.* Jaipur: Prateeksha Publications.

Viswanath, K. (2008). Perspectives on Models of Interpersonal Health Behavior. In K. Glanz, B. K. Rimer & K. Viswanath (Eds.) *Health Behavior and Health Education. Theory, Research, and Practice*. (4th ed.) San Francisco, CA: Jossey-Bass, pp. 271-281.

Wallington, S. F. (2014). Health Disparities Research and Practice. The Role of Language and Health Communication. In H. E. Hamilton & W. S. Chou (Eds.) *The Routledge Handbook of Language and Health Communication*. London-New York: Routledge, pp.168-183.

Warren, J. T. & Fassett, D. L. (2011). *Communication. A Critical/Cultural Introduction*. Los Angeles-London-New Delhi-Singapore-Washington DC: Sage Publications, Inc.

Weinstein, N. D., Sandman, P. M., & Blalock, S. J. (2008). The Precaution Adoption Process Model. In K. Glanz, B. K. Rimer & K. Viswanath (Eds.) *Health Behavior and Health Education. Theory, Research, and Practice* (4th ed.) San Francisco, CA: Jossey-Bass, pp. 123-147.

Welch Cline, R. J. (2003). Everyday Interpersonal Communication and Health. In T. L. Thompson, A. Dorsey, K. I. Miller, R. Parrott (Eds.) *Handbook of Health Communication*. New York-London: Lawrence Erlbaum Associates., pp.285-313.

Wellin, E. (1977). Theoretical Orientations in Medical Anthropology. In D. Landy (Ed.) *Culture, Disease, and Healing: Studies in Medical Anthropology*. New York: Macmillan.

Wermuth, L. (2003). *Global Inequality and Human Needs*. Boston: Pearson Education, Inc.

WHO (1946). Constitution of the World Health Organisation. International health conference; 1946, New York.

Wickrama, K. A. S., Lorenz, F. O., Conger, R. D. & Elder, G. H. (1997). Linking Occupational Conditions to Physical Health through Material, Social and Interpersonal Processes. *Journal of Health and Social Behavior*. 38 (4): 363-375.

Wilkinson, R. & Pickett, K. (2009). *The Spirit Level: Why Equality is Better for Everyone*. London: Allen Lane.

Wilkinson, R. G. (1997). Health Inequalities: Relative or Absolute Material Standards? *British Medical Journal*, 314(7080), pp. 591-595.

Williams, D. R. (1990). Socioeconomic Differntials in Health: A Review and Redirection. *Social Psychology Quarterly* 53 (2): 81-99.

Williams, G. G. (2002). Improving Patient's Health Through Supporting the Autonomy of Patients and Providers. In E. L. Deci & R. M. Ryan (Eds.) *Handbook of Self-Determination Research*. Rochester, NY: the University of Rochester Press, pp. 233-254.

World Bank Group (2015). *World Development Report. Mind, Society, and Behavior*. Washington D.C: International Bank for Reconstruction and Development/ The World Bank.

World Health Organization Regional Office for Europe (2013). *A European Policy Framework and Strategy for the 21st Century*. Cohenhagen: World Health Organization (WHO) Regional Office for Europe.

World Health Organization Regional Office for Europe (2013). *Health 2020. A European Policy Framework and Strategy for the 21st Century*. WHO Regional Office for Europe: Denmark.

Yach, D. & Beaglehole, R. (2004). Globalization of Risks for Chronic Diseases Demands Global Solutions. In R. L. Harris & M. Seid (eds.) *Globalization and Health*. Leiden & Boston: Brill, pp. 213-233.

Yach, D. (2006). Chronic Disease. In B. S. Levy & V. W. Sidel (eds.) *Social Injustice and Public Health*. Oxford-New York: Oxford University Press, pp. 253-276.

Websites

About.com 2015
1). About.com 2015 a
http://psychology.about.com/od/historyofpsychology/a/psychistory.htm, accessed on April 9th, 2015.
2). About.com 2015 b
http://webtrends.about.com/od/web20/a/what-is-web-30.htm, accessed on November 2nd, 2015.
BBC news services 2014
http://www.bbc.com/news/health-25635121, accessed on June 18th, 2015.
Bulletin of the World Health Organization 2008
http://www.who.int/bulletin/volumes/86/12/08-021208/en/, accessed on June 15th, 2015.
Centers for Disease Control and Prevention (CDC)
1). CDC 2010
http://www.cdc.gov/h1n1flu/cdcresponse.htm, accessed on September 3rd, 2015.
2). CDC 2014 a
http://www.cdc.gov/teenpregnancy/about/index.htm, accessed on June 22nd, 2015.
3). CDC 2014 b
http://www.cdc.gov/flu/avianflu/h7n9-virus.htm, accessed on July 22nd, 2015.
4). CDC 2015
http://www.cdc.gov/coronavirus/mers/index.html, accessed on September 4th, 2015.
Ebizmba.com 2016
http://www.ebizmba.com/articles/social-networking-websites, accessed on January 20th, 2016.
Emedicinehealth.com 2015
1). Emedicinehealth.com 2015 a
http://www.emedicinehealth.com/mad_cow_disease_and_variant_creutzfeldt-jakob/page2_em.htm, accessed on September 4th, 2015.
2). Emedicinehealth.com 2015 b
http://www.emedicinehealth.com/checkup/article_em.htm#a_checkup_how_often, accessed on November 1st, 2015.
EndocrineWeb 2015
http://www.endocrineweb.com/conditions/type-1-diabetes/what-insulin, accessed on September 5th, 2015.
IGI-Global 2015
http://www.igi-global.com/dictionary/positivist-epistemology/23062, accessed on April 9th, 2015).
IMedia Connection 2015
http://www.imediaconnection.com/content/34206.asp, accessed on November 2nd, 2015.
International Agency for Research on Cancer (IARC, WHO, 2013)

http://www.iarc.fr/en/media-centre/iarcnews/pdf/pr221_E.pdf, accessed on September 12th, 2015.

MedicineNet.com 2015
http://www.medicinenet.com/aerobic_exercise/article.htm, accessed on September 5th, 2015.

MediLexicon International, Ltd. 2014
http://www.medicalnewstoday.com/articles/154874.php, accessed on April 9th, 2015).

NASA 2015
http://climate.nasa.gov/effects/, accessed on September 15th, 2015.

National Geographic 2015
http://environment.nationalgeographic.com/environment/global-warming/ozone-depletion-overview/depletion-overview/, accessed on September 15th, 2015.

News.softpedia.com 2007
http://news.softpedia.com/news/Top-10-Infectious-Diseases-That-Have-Killed-Most-People-70741.shtml, accessed on January 29th, 2016.

Northbound Treatment Services 2013
http://www.livingsober.com/affluenza-drug-addiction/#.VYZyxPmqqko, accessed on June 19th, 2015.

O'Reilly Media Inc. (2015)
http://www.oreilly.com/pub/a/web2/archive/what-is-web-20.html, accessed on November 2nd, 2015.

PCWorld 2015
http://www.pcworld.com/article/143110/article.html, accessed on November 2nd, 2015.

PsychCentral 2015
http://psychcentral.com/lib/obesity-and-mental-health/, accessed on September 11th, 2015.

Public Broadcasting Services (PBS)
1). PBS 2014
http://www.pbs.org/newshour/updates/diseases-thought-eradicated-reappear-u-s/, accessed on September 4th, 2015.
2). PBS 2015 a
http://www.pbs.org/wgbh/pages/frontline/sickaroundtheworld/countries/models.html, accessed on June 24th, 2015
3). PBS 2015 b
http://www.pbs.org/wgbh/pages/frontline/sickaroundtheworld/, accessed June 24, 2015.

Sex and Drugs and Rock and Health.com n.d.
http://www.sexanddrugsandrockandhealth.com/page3.htm, accessed on April 16th, 2015.

Sociology 2009
http://sociology-4-all.blogspot.hk/2009/03/auguste-comte-1798-1857-founding-father.html, accessed on April 9th, 2015.

Study.com 2015
http://study.com/academy/lesson/etic-and-emic-world-views-in-anthropology.html, accessed on October 14th, 2015.

TechTarget 2015
http://whatis.techtarget.com/definition/crowdsource-testing, accessed on November 2nd, 2015.

The College of Physicians of Philadelphia 2015
http://www.historyofvaccines.org/content/articles/disease-eradication, accessed on July 22nd, 2015.
The Medical Journal of Australia 2004
https://www.mja.com.au/journal/2004/180/4/globalisation-what-it-and-how-does-it-affect-health, accessed on July 19th, 2015.
U.S. Environmental Protection Agency (EPA)
1). EPA 1991
http://www.epa.gov/iaq/pdfs/sick_building_factsheet.pdf, accessed on September 12th, 2015.
2). EPA2013
http://www.epa.gov/wastes/hazard/tsd/pcbs/pubs/about.htm, accessed on September 9th, 2015.
3). EPA 2015
http://www.epa.gov/climatechange/ghgemissions/gases.html, accessed on September 15th, 2015.
WebMD
1). WebMD 2013
http://www.webmd.com/brain/mad-cow-disease-basics?page=3#1, accessed on September 4th, 2015.
2). WebMD 2015 a
http://www.webmd.com/sleep-disorders/features/important-sleep-habits?page=2, accessed on September 11th, 2015.
3). WebMD 2015 b
http://www.webmd.com/diabetes/guide/insulin-resistance-syndrome, accessed on June 22nd, 2015.
Wellness city.co.th 2015
https://www.youtube.com/watch?v=poS-t_nYFrE, accessed on January 23rd, 2016.
World Health Organization (WHO)
1). WHO 2014 a
http://www.who.int/mediacentre/news/releases/2014/world-health-statistics-2014/en/, accessed on June 19th, 2015.
2). WHO 2014 b
http://www.who.int/topics/emerging_diseases/en/, accessed on January 29th, 2016.
3). WHO 2015 a (non communicable disease)
http://www.who.int/mediacentre/factsheets/fs355/en/, accessed Jan 11th, 2015.
4). WHO 2015 b antimicrobial drug resistance
http://www.who.int/csr/disease/OP_AMR_FINAL.pdf?ua=1, accessed on July 22nd, 2015.
5).WHO 2015 c top ten cause of death
http://who.int/mediacentre/factsheets/fs310/en/index1.html, accessed on September 4th, 2015.
6). WHO 2015 d
http://www.who.int/tb/people_and_communities/advocacy_communication/en/, accessed October 22nd, 2015.
7). WHO 2015 e dengue and severe dengue

http://www.who.int/mediacentre/factsheets/fs117/en/, accessed on Jan 17th, 2016.
8). WHO 2016
http://www.who.int/topics/emerging_diseases/en/, accessed on January 29th, 2016.
Yourdictionary.com 2015
1). Yourdictionary.com 2015 a
http://www.yourdictionary.com/phenotype, accessed on November 16th, 2015.
2). Yourdictionary.com 2015 b
http://www.yourdictionary.com/genotype, accessed on November 16th, 2015.

About the Author

Patchanee Malikhao, Ph.D.
HIV/AIDS Sociologist,
Health Communication & Communication
for Sustainability Specialist
Fecund Communication
pmalikhao@gmail.com

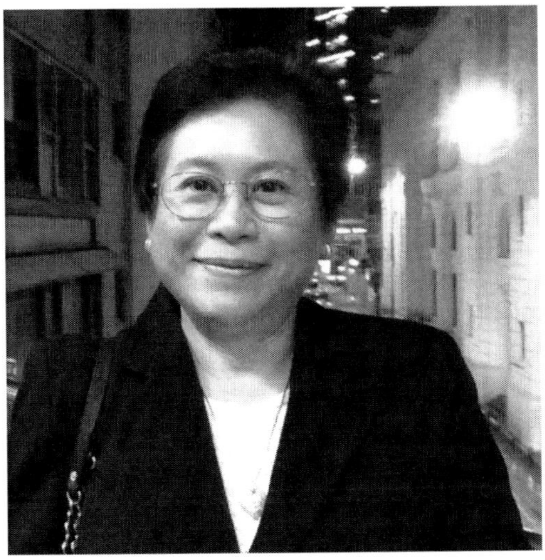

Dr. Patchanee Malikhao is a Sociologist with competencies in mass communication research and graphic arts research. She has a variety of research interests ranging from communication for sustainable social change, over health related areas such as HIV/AIDS. She is also interested in mindful journalism, Buddhism and social communication, globalization and culture, intercultural communi-cation, Thai culture and communi-cation.

She has worked and received special training as a tutor, lecturer, instructor, researcher, and she is also a writer in the fields of Communication for Social Change, Health Communication, research and development in digital media, and sociology of the media, culture, and communication in the Netherlands, Belgium, Australia, the US, Hong Kong, and Thailand, her home country.

She received a Ph.D. in Sociology from the University of Queensland, Australia; a Master of Science in Printing Technology (currently called Print Media) from the Rochester Institute of Technology (RIT) in Rochester, New York; a Master of Arts in Mass Communication from the Faculty of Journalism and Mass Communication, Thammasat University, Bangkok, Thailand; and a Bachelor of Science (Hons.) in Photographic Science and Printing Technology from Chulalongkorn University, Bangkok, Thailand.

She was a recipient of a Fulbright Scholarship, the Australian Postgraduate Award Scholarship, and a distinguished award in printing studies from the Tab Nilanidhi Foundation, Thailand.

Index

E

F

G

H

I

K

L

T

U

W

Z